Simple Keto Meal Prep

Complete Guide with Life-changing Ketogenic Foods for Beginners and Advanced Users

By Steven Jack

Disclaimer

Disclaimer and Terms of Use: Effort has been made to ensure that the information in this book is accurate and complete, however, the author and the publisher do not warrant the accuracy of the information, text and graphics contained within the book due to the rapidly changing nature of science, research, known and unknown facts and internet. The Author and the publisher do not hold any responsibility for errors, omissions or contrary interpretation of the subject matter herein. This book is presented solely for motivational and informational purposes only.

Table of Contents

Introduction

Losing your weight and keeping it under control is perhaps one of the main concern of individuals these days! Especially given the obesity rates are at an all-time high, which is further causing the rate of health diseases to rise up!

Even though there are hundreds and perhaps thousands of diets out there! Very few of them are actually effective.

But even fewer are as effective as the Ketogenic Diet!

What is the heart of this diet you ask?

Well, the main objective is to simply cut down your carbs and refrain yourself from eating food and ingredients such as flour, sweets, cereals and potatoes! If you do things right, not only will your health improve, but you will see a significant reduction in your weight!

This happens primarily because, when you push carbs out of your system, your body enters a state of Ketosis, which encourages your body to burn your fat to get its required energy. This accelerates the whole fat burning process and turns your body into a literal fat burning machine!

Several years ago, lots of people believed that low-carb diets were actually fads, but those misconceptions are now being discredited as researchers and scientists are coming to a conclusion that low carb weight loss regimes such as the Keto diet, is actually the safest and most effective diet to go for!

Throughout the pages of this book, you will find extremely detailed information regarding the basic concepts of Ketogenic Diet as well as Meal Prepping!

So, if you lead a busy life, you will still be able to stick to your Keto diet with ease, thanks to the amazing Meal Prepping ideas found in this book.

Once you are done with the intro, feel free to dive into the plethora of amazing Keto friendly recipes and experiment until you find the best plan that suits your needs!

Part 1: Keto Made Easy

Chapter 1: Ketogenic Diet Basics

Looking at the history of Ketogenic Diet

Ketogenic Diet has a origin that goes way back to the 1900s.
Even at that time, there were lots of different "Wannabe" diets that were trying to get a chunk of the market! However, during 1942, Ketogenic Diet came into the scene and completely revolutionized the whole spectrum.
This is a regime that was meticulously created by one Dr. Russell Wilder, who at that time was working at the Mayo Clinic.
It should be noted though that the original aim behind the conception of this diet was not to deal with weight loss, rather, Russell created the diet in hopes of experimenting with patients and finding a cure for those who were suffering from epilepsy.
Interested to know how the diet worked?
Well, it simply removes or greatly lowered down the amount of carbohydrate intake!
Most of the foods which we eat nowadays include junk foods and another oily produces which are jam-packed with a bucket load of carbohydrates which ultimately leads us to gain more weight than we had hoped for.
The main goal of a Ketogenic Diet is to lower down the level of Carbohydrate intake and improve the condition of your body by encouraging it to burn down more fat instead of glucose to obtain the necessary energy for daily activates.
If that sounds a little bit confusing to you right now, don't worry as all confusions will go away as you go through the introductory pages of this book.

What exactly is Ketogenic Diet?

So, you are well versed on the history of the diet! But you must be wondering, what exactly is a "Ketogenic Diet" right?
Well, we all know that our body requires energy for proper functioning right? It uses carbohydrates, protein and fats as the most common sources of energy.
However, due to exposing ourselves for a really long time to a diet that focused on low fat and high carbohydrates, we have become used to depending on glucose (coming from carbohydrates) as the main source of energy.

As long as glucose is in our body, the body will always opt to use glucose as its primary source of energy. It is only when the level of carbohydrates is depleted from our body, the body starts to look for other sources of energy, namely, fat!

The bottom line then? If you simply cut down your carbohydrate intake, your body will burn more and more fat to power its cells and organs! Improving your rate at which you burn your fat.

So, to summarize, the primary aim of Ketogenic diet is to essentially convert your body into a literal fat burning machine!

This diet is packed with a plethora of benefits that are discussed in a later chapter, but just to give you an idea:

- It will help you control your appetite
- It will improve your mental clarity
- It will lower down inflammation in your body
- It will improve the stability of your blood sugar levels
- It will eliminate the risk of heart burn
- It forces your body burn fat as energy instead of carbs
- And most importantly, it does wonders for weight loss

As mentioned, the effects mentioned above are just some of the few amazing benefits a person will enjoy after embarking on a Ketogenic diet.

And just in case you are wondering, a Ketogenic diet consists of meals that are designed to be low on carbohydrate with moderate levels of protein and high fat contents.

These are also known as the "Macronutrients".

And to go deeper into the topic, A Ketogenic Diet encourages your body into a state of "Ketosis".

This is what we are going to discuss next.

So, what exactly is Ketosis?

As you can already tell, "Ketosis" is the key word here.

So, when you start to deprive your body of carbohydrates, the body begins to automatically seek out other sources that it can use to obtain the required energy. Since fat is present in abundance in our body, it immediately turns its attention to burning down fat.

Whenever carbohydrates are not readily available, the liver starts t break down fat into fatty acids, which are further broken down into energy-rich substances known as "Ketones."

This whole process is known as Ketosis!

Looking deeply into Ketones

Once your body decides that it is time to start burning fat, the body takes the fat to the liver where it is broken down into glycerol and fatty acids through a process known as Beta-Oxidation.
These fatty acids are broken down to even further smaller molecules through a process of Ketogenesis, which leads to the creation of a very specific ketone known as acetoacetate.
Given enough time, the body slowly starts to completely adapt itself to use these ketones as a source of energy, and the muscles learn to convert the acetoacetate into Beta-Hydroxybutyrate (BHB for short), which is the body's preferred Ketogenic source of energy for the brain.
Asides from that, acetone is also produced, which the body expels as waste.
The glycerol created during the beta-oxidation goes through a process known as gluconeogenesis that converts the glycerol into glucose that the body uses for energy.
Alternatively, the excess protein obtained during a Keto diet is also utilized for energy by converting them to Glucose.
This allows the body to satisfy the minimum need of Glucose of the body without actually using carbohydrates to get it!

Symptoms to know that you are on Ketosis

If you are a newcomer, then it might be difficult for you to tell whether your body has entered into a state of Ketosis or not.
The following are rules of thumb to help you detect if your body is indeed in Ketosis.

- Your mouth will feel dry, and you feel have increased thirst
- The number of washroom visits will increase as you might need to urinate more often.
- Your breath will have a slight "Fruity" smell to it that will resemble that of a nail polish
- Aside from those three, you will get the sensation mentioned above of having a low hunger level and increased physical energy.

What are macronutrients to control?

The main macronutrients that you should consider when on a Ketogenic diet are the proteins, fats and carbs.

You would be astonished to know just how much we lie to ourselves and how many carbs we tend to unknowingly consume on a daily basis.

Tracing macros will help you to improve the effectiveness of your Keto diet and accelerate the rate at which you lose weight.

You can bring about a greater control over your diet if you know your macros. When you are tracking your macros, make sure to consider the grams instead of the percentages.

To give you a breakdown of the three macros

- **Protein:** These are also known as the building blocks of our body since they help to generate and heal a different kind of tissues in our body. They promote growth and development.
- **Fat:** While people often look at Fat in a negative way, these are also essential as they act as a backup reservoir of energy for the body.
- **Carbohydrates:** Carbohydrates are the primary source of energy in our body. They range from simple to complex and are often very easily converted to energy.

How these macronutrients are providing energy to your body?

The cells in our body need a constant supply of energy in order to stay alive and active. Even if you are not doing anything at all, your body is in a constant state of generating energy in order to keep you breathing.

However, as the energy conservation law dictates, energy cannot be created or destroyed. Rather, it is simply converted from one form to another.

In case of your body, it also needs to get the energy it requires from somewhere right?

Well, this is where you the concept of macro nutrients will come into play.

The body is able to actually obtain energy from the above mentioned macro nutrients through a very complex biochemical process.

Having a basic understanding of this process is essential for you to properly science behind a Ketogenic Diet.

So, let's break down how the body breaks down the three macros to get energy.

From Protein

Protein is quite possibly the least preferred macronutrient when it comes to supplying the body with energy.

This is primarily due to the fact that protein is generally reserved to be used for other function than providing the body with energy.

Proteins provide structural support to every cell in the body and help it to properly maintain and regulate the body tissues.

To be more exact, proteins tend to act as enzymes that play a crucial role in the biochemical reactions of our body. Without these enzymes acting as catalysts, the essential reactions of our body won't work or will be dramatically slowed down.

This means, the body won't be able to metabolize or digest properly.

Aside from that, proteins also help to maintain the fluid and acid-base balance of our body, which allows the body to transport oxygen throughout the internal system and pass out waste.

Just in case you are wondering about the structure of Protein! They are made of up tiny parts known as Amino Acids.

Whenever you eat proteins, the body slowly starts to break them down into individual amino acids, which are later converted into sugar through a process known as deamination.

If needed, then the body is able to use these converted amino acids for energy. But this means that less protein would be available for other bodily functions, therefore this process is generally avoided.

From Carbohydrates

Even though your body is designed to utilize any food for energy, it always prefers to go for carbohydrate first!

Whenever you are consuming carbohydrate, they are broken down into glucose, which is one of easiest molecule available for energy.

Glucose is absorbed through the walls of your small intestine where it enters the body through your bloodstream, causing the blood glucose level to rise.

This glucose causes the pancreas to send out insulin, which picks up the sugar from the blood steam and carry them to the cells to be used as energy.

Once the cells have used up the glucose it requires, the rest of the glucose is converted into glycogen, which is then stored in muscles or livers.

You should understand now that the liver has a very limited ability to store glycogen. The extra glucose that aren't converted, are converted into triglycerides, which is a form of fat.

From Fat

The body starts to look towards fat for energy when carbohydrates aren't readily available.

The fat you eat is broken down into their small components known as fatty acids, which enters the blood steam as well through the walls of your small intestine.

Most cells can directly use fatty acids for energy but some of the more specialized cells present in your muscles and brain can't utilize fatty acids directly. To fulfill the needs of these cells, the body starts to utilize the fatty acids to create ketones.

How to keep your body in Ketosis?

While following the natural guidelines of the Ketogenic Diet will let you enter a state of Ketosis just fine, there are certain steps that you can take in order to further enhance the effectiveness of your Ketosis.

- Always make sure to keep your daily carb intake below 20 carbs
- Keep your protein levels at around 70g per day
- Make sure not to starve! Make sure to consume adequate levels of fat and remember that you need fat to burn fat.
- Always make sure to avoid snacking and stick to breakfast, lunch and dinner as your meal plans

What are some of the unwanted effects of Ketogenic diet?

Just like any other diet, it is very much possible that during the early days of your Ketogenic Diet, you might experience some minor discomfort due to the major changes that your body is going through.
Don't worry as these symptoms will eventually go away within a week or two.
Common symptoms include:

- Mental fogginess
- Headaches
- Keto-Flu
- Aggravation
- Dizziness

Ketosis causes your body to lose a good amount of electrolytes, which is one of the main reason as to why you might experience those symptoms.
The best way to deal with these is to replace the lost electrolytes by drinking more water.
Asides from that, the ones mentioned above, there are a few more factors that you should keep in mind such as:

- Frequent desire to urinate
- Hypoglycemia
- Constipation
- Increased Sugar Craving
- Diarrhea
- Sleep problem

Chapter 2: Understanding the different variations of Keto diet

If you are done with the last chapter, then by now you should have a pretty clear grasp of the concept of Ketogenic Diet.
Let me take you further into the different types of Ketogenic diet now.
Surprised?
Well, not every single plan is suitable for everyone right?
Every individual is different and the needs and requirements varies from one person to the next.
There are some people who have specific limitations and are unable to break that limitation, because otherwise, things would go south for them.
Those limitations force them to consume more carbohydrate than the specified daily margin.
So, are they supposed to give up on their dreams of ever following a Keto diet? Not really!
The whole regime of a Ketogenic Diet has been designed to be extremely versatile and provides a very flexible foundation, which can be modified very easily in order to meet the requirements of people with special needs.
Generally speaking, there are three different types of Ketogenic diet at present.

- Standard Ketogenic Diet (STD)
- Targeted Ketogenic Diet (TKD)
- Cyclic Ketogenic Diet (CKD)

Each type of diet is suitable for a specific group of people. I will be breaking them down one by one for your convenience.

The Standard Ketogenic Diet or (STD)

Suitable for: Normal individuals with no disease of   limitation other than the want of losing their weight.
Ketogenic Ratios: 5% Carb; 75% Fat; 20% Protein
This is the most widely followed type of Diet and this generally requires only a single rule to be followed.
Simply put, try to eat as fewer carbs as possible throughout the day.
This type of the diet is often compared to a segment of another diet known as "Induction" phase of the Atkins diet.
To help you understand the similarity, here is a brief overview of the induction phase.

First Phase of Atkins: The first phase of the Atkins Diet is known as the "Induction" phase.

In this phase, you are essentially needed to cut out the maximum amount of carbohydrates from your daily diet.

As a rule of thumb, you are to bring down your carb intake to just 20g per day, which should primarily come from vegetables.

As for proteins, you may go for fish, shellfish, eggs and poultry.

And most definitely refrain yourself from baked goods, alcohol, grain and pasta.

For your STD, the Carb count is also required to be kept around 20-50 grams per day. The exact amount may vary a little, but it should never go beyond 50 grams.

Cyclic Ketogenic Diet (CKD)

Suitable for: This diet is essential for those individuals who are closely related to Body Building and heavy workouts. In fact, this diet has been often called to be the "Perfect Body Building Diet".

With this diet, you will be able to build your muscle without gaining fat and inject your body with anabolic hormones without the use of any artificial supplements.

Ketogenic Ratios: This plan will simply require you to undergo a period of high-carb session that is to be preceded by a normal Ketogenic session.

For example, you might follow a very strict Ketogenic diet (low carb) for 5 days a week, and then go for a high carb feeding for the next 2 days.

The Cyclical Diet or shortly called "CKD" basically indicates a cycling period that rounds between sessions of diet with high protein, low carb and high fat which are followed by sessions of high protein, high carb and obviously low at.

During the majority of the time, you will be going through the standard rules of a Keto diet, and during the rest, you are expose yourself to a high carb diet.

The process keeps on moving in a cyclic order, hence the name.

As much weird as the whole process might sound, there is actually a very sound scientific reasoning behind this process, which enhances the productivity and effectiveness of any body building regime.

To make things short and simple, the most importance aspect of the diet is that it helps to increase the serum level of multiple hormones of our body (usually the ones that are related to promoting physical body growth).

These hormones include

- Certain Growth Hormones
- Testosterone
- IGF-1

But now, you might be wondering, how does one initiate this form of diet?

Well, as mentioned in the ratio section of the diet, the Cyclical Diet will only require you to consume high levels of fat, protein and low levels of carbohydrates, which is then to be followed by periods of high protein, high carb and low fat.

Keep in mind that there are multiple variations of CKD, but the one that I mentioned here is the most suitable one body building.

Targeted Ketogenic Diet (TKD)

Suitable for: This diet is recommended for those people who are interested in body building/ or are weight lifters but are unable to follow CKD due to medical or health complications. This regime gives a boost of energy to promote muscle growth and might give an additional rep or two.

Ketogenic Ratios: The carb intake of this regime largely depends on the level of workout.

TKD is a much more refined version of the Simple Ketogenic Diet to be exact.

Simply put, TKD will require you to eat carbs about 30-60 minutes before going into a session of heavy exercise.

This has been looked upon as being more of a combination of both a Standard Ketogenic Diet and Cyclical Ketogenic Diet which ultimately allows you to perform activities which may put an incredible amount of strain on your body.

Keep in mind though that a Cyclical Keto Diet might be more suitable for advanced body builders or Keto Athletes.

TKD is more suitable for people who are in their beginning/intermediate phase.

However, one thing to keep in mind while following a TKD is to only go for produces that are packed with digestible carbohydrates. In short, go for produces that have a high Glycemic index. This will help you to avoid stomach disorders.

Other foods which you might want to avoid during this diet might include high fructose based foods as they might allow the liver to replenish glycogen, which is unacceptable for a Keto Diet.

This diet works following a very simple theory. Since you are consuming a large amount of High-Carb food before working out, the carbs get burned out right away while working! This will automatically return you to a state of Ketosis in no time!

Another tip would be to try and avoid fatty foods right after your training period, otherwise it may impair the nutrient absorption and hamper a proper recovery of muscles.

With the information provided above, you should have a good idea of which variation of Ketogenic Diet is the best on for you!

However, there are still certain factors that you should keep in mind. In case of the following scenarios, it is highly advised against following a Ketogenic Diet.

Who should avoid the Ketogenic diet?

- Individuals who are suffering from Gallbladder disease or have no Gallbladder should refrain from following Ketogenic diet

- Individuals who have undergone a gastric bypass/ weight loss surgery should avoid Ketogenic Diet

- Individuals who are suffering from various metabolic disorders should stay away from Ketogenic diet as it might hamper the metabolic processes further

- Pregnant women as well breastfeeding women should refrain themselves from a Keto diet because they require a much higher protein count

- People who are suffering from pancreatic issues should avoid the diet as well

- People with kidney stones should avoid it as well

- People with a BMI of less than 20 should stay away from Keto diets as well as additional loss of weight might be harmful to them

- People with anorexia are also required to avoid the diet as the psychological fear of gaining weight will eventually force them to avoid eating the proper levels of fat altogether. This might eventually lead to some very severe consequences.

Chapter 3: Top benefits of Ketogenic Diet

A Ketogenic diet won't only keep you healthy, but it comes with a plethora of amazing benefits as well!

Some of the major ones that you should know about are listed below for your convenience.

Improved Sleep Cycle: If you adopt the Ketogenic diet properly, then you will enjoy a more sound sleep. Many Keto followers have reported that they were able to get a proper sleep without any interruption whatsoever. These improvements are strongly linked to the fact that you are limiting your daily glucose intake, which tends to facilitated lower levels of chronic inflammation in your body, which further allows your body to stay in a deep rest.

Improved Digestion: If you shift to a Keto diet by lowering down your sugar and carb intake, it will improve your digestion and your gut health. This is also closely linked to low grain consumption that usually leads to bloating or feelings of indigestions.

Improve mood: The production of Ketones in your body are beneficial when it comes to stabilizing and controlling your neurotransmitters such as serotonin or dopamine. The stabilization of these neurotransmitters helps to improve your mood and clarify your thoughts.

Will keep you energized: Ketones are a much more reliable energy source for your body and it will keep you feeling energized for the whole day. Chronic fatigue symptoms that you might be experiencing will soon go away and you will feel more energetic.

Since you are cutting down your reliance on using carbs as a source of energy, your body will also be spared of "Sugar Rush" effect where your body gets brief surges of "energy" followed by a prolonged period of fatigue.

If your body is using Ketones as the energy source, your body will constantly stay fueled due to the abundance of fat present in your body.

It will help you fight lots of diseases: The different forms of Ketogenic Diet have been seen to have the potential to tackle various diseases such as Alzheimer's, polycystic ovary syndrome, depression,   traumatic brain injury, stoke alongside various other diseases that have been plaguing our generation.

There are many studies conducted by various reputable institutions that have shown significantly positive outcomes from following a Ketogenic diet.

Caner is also one of the diseases that have been receiving significant positive results when linked to Ketogenic Diet, as it is seen that is able to "Starve" cancerous cells.

The original notion of starving cancer cells is not new though ,as it was brought in 1942 by a German Scientists named Otto Warburg, who proposed an idea where he said that the prime caused of cancer was the fermentation of sugar within out body cells.

To tackle this notion, the main action was to remove or significantly decline sugar consumption.

Since Ketogenic diet aims to do exactly that, it acts as a strong agent against Cancer.

Improved Weight Loss: Lowering down your card intake is one of the most effective way to cut down weight. This has been to "Go-To" strategy for individuals since the later 1800s, ever since people started to trim down your body weight.

There have been several randomized and controlled clinical trials on the turn of the century that proves the efficacy of a low – carb diet when it comes to dealing improving weight loss.

By preventing the accumulation of sugar in your body, Ketogenic diets drive down insulin production that compels your body to use up your stored fat.

This also works ,even when your body is sleeping! It will keep on burning fat to satisfy its energy needs.

The effects might be slow, but you will definitely notice positive effects!

It will help you control your appetite: The ability to actually be in control of your hunger and manage it accordingly is extremely empowering.

Hunger is perhaps one of the most difficult feelings to control for an individual trying to follow a diet. If you are unable to control your hunger, you will eat more and your dietary efforts will go in vain.

This is also one of the primary reason as to why many individuals give up following a diet hallway through.

Ketogenic Diet on the other hand helps to lower down your hunger and food cravings and keep you feeling full.

Fat is an extremely satisfying and fulfilling nutrient that helps you to reduce your appetite alongside ketones.

In fact, while on a Ketogenic Diet, you might even go through times when you won't experience the desire to eat at all!

It will help you to effortlessly maintain optimal weight: If your body is adapted to a Keto diet, it will basically mean that your body has turned into a mean big fat burning machine!

This means that the amount of effort that you would need put to maintain your optimal physique and body weight will be significantly reduced, as your body will keep burning fat throughout the day.

This also applies to physical activities such as exercises as well! The fat burning mode of your body will further enhance the effectiveness of your daily exercise and physical activities.

Your body will start to use fat as its fuel: I have already discussed this earlier, but even so! This has to be brought up as an advantage.

When your body adapts itself to Keto diet, it will go into a state of Ketosis where your body will recognize fat as its primary source of energy.

This is generating Ketone Body's for fuel and burn more and more fat!

It helps to regulated insulin levels : Insulin is needed by our bodies as it facilitates the blood sugar levels. Insulin acts as a kind of messenger between glucose and our body cells, letting it know when to start using glucose as a source of energy.

While you are on a higher carb diet, your body will essentially experience more insulin spikes every time your blood sugar level rises.

Nutritional Ketosis helps to facilitate the reduction of insulin levels because of your lower blood sugar levels through lowered consumption of carbs.

Helps to deal with various metabolic syndromes: Metabolic Syndrome refers to a type of medical condition that increase the risk of your suffering from heart diseases or diabetes.

Some syndromes include:

- Abdominal obesity
- High blood pressure
- Low HDL cholesterol levels
- High triglycerides
- High blood sugar levels

All of the above mentioned symptoms can be easily managed by following a Ketogenic diet.

Chapter 4: Common mistakes while following a Ketogenic Diet

We are human beings, and regardless of how much versed we are on a particular topic, we are still bound to make a few mistakes every now and then. So, before you jump into the Keto diet! You should be aware of the following most common mistakes that people seem to make during their early Keto days.

Not having a proper meal plan: This is one of the biggest mistakes people make when trying to embark on the diet! Those who do not make a proper meal plan often end up failing to control themselves because they are always hungry. It might take some time to prepare a meal plan, but it's nothing impossible! Meal Planning will save you from the headaches and frustrations, but will also act as fantastic way to save money!

Missing out on your electrolytes: Electrolytes are extremely essential in an Ketogenic diet and are necessary for this particular diet as well. If you don't consume Vitamin D, magnesium, sodium, potassium and salt, you might experience various negative symptoms such as lethargy, constipation and fatigue. These are often known as "Keto-Flu". This is one of the reason as to why many people tend to quit the diet!

Comparing yourself to others: This is a very big mistake that people seem to make! Just stop comparing yourself to others! You should learn to appreciate the fact that every one's body reacts differently to dietary changes and some people progress faster while others progress slower. It is pointless to compare yourself to others and feel disheartened. At the end of the day, you will achieve your goal, you just have to wait for it.

Not getting proper sleep: Just like water, your body requires a good amount of sleep otherwise it will fall into a state of fatigue, making you feel lethargic all throughout the day.

Not drinking enough water: Without drinking a good amount of water, your body won't be able to properly do what it's supposed to do! You have to drink more water than you used to during a Keto diet in order to ensure that your whole body is working properly. A general rule of thumb is to drink at least 0.5 to 1 ounces of water per pound of your body weight per day.

Not being flexible enough: Following a Ketogenic diet, or even any diet for that matter would basically mean that you will have to change many of your previous habits in order to appreciate your new diet plan. Some people often fail to bend their personal rules and end up not being able to follow the diet properly! Try to create a strong mental picture before going into the diet to ensure that everything goes smoothly.

Losing patience: Before you decide to jump into the Ketogenic Diet, you should have a good understanding that since you have been running on carbohydrates your whole life, and all of a sudden shifting your diet will require some time for your body to habituate itself to. So, don't be impatient!

Chapter 5: Tips for a Successful Keto Diet

The following tips will help you to improve the effectiveness of your Ketogenic diet even further!

- Make sure to go through your pantry and get rid of all high carb ingredients and foods before starting your Keto journey

- Try to follow the Ketogenic diet with a friend or another family member. It will help you stay encourage and inspired all throughout the journey

- Make sure to eat sufficient amount of food and maintaining the levels of fat, protein and carbs as needed

- Try to make dishes that you will actually enjoy! Being on a diet might be difficult if you are not actually enjoying it. There are a plethora of recipes that you can choose for your Ketogenic diet, so make your meal plan accordingly.

- Try to maintain a check list or something similar to track your progress

- Make sure to keep your sodium intake in check to avoid future problems during your Ketogenic journey. Easy steps may include
    - ✓ Drinking organic broth if possible
    - ✓ Taking a just a pinch of pink salt with you consumed meals
    - ✓ Adding about ¼ teaspoon of pink salt to 16 ounces of water consumed
    - ✓ Adding vegetables such as kelp to your dishes
    - ✓ Eating up vegetables such as cucumber or celery for a more natural approach to sodium replenishment

- It is essential to maintain a proper exercise routine to make sure that your body is in tip-top shape all throughout the regime.

- Try to buy a counter to keep track of your carbs

- Make sure to keep yourself packed with a good amount of water to replenish flushed electrolytes

Chapter 6: Frequently Asked Questions

More and more people and discovering their way into the Ketogenic diet every single day! And for absolute new comers, the transition might seem a little difficult.

If you are a new comer as well, this brief section will help you to answer some of the most frequently asked questions that people have regarding this particular diet.

How should you track your carb intake?

The most generic way to track carb intake is to use the services of MyFitnessPal alongside their apps. You cannot track net carbs with this app though, but it will help you to track your overall carbohydrate intake and fiber intake. To calculate your net carbs, simply deduce the total fiber intake from your total carb intake.

How long does it usually take to get into Ketosis?

A Ketogenic diet plan isn't a diet that can simply push you immediately into Ketosis! It's a slow and gradual process that takes time to work properly. You won't enter Ketosis until your body has adjusted itself to the new diet, only after which you will enter Ketosis.

This usually takes somewhere between 2-7 days depending on your body type, activity levels and the food that you are consuming.

Perhaps the fastest and easier way to enter Ketosis is to simply follow the Keto food guidelines and limit your carb intake to less than 20g per day.

Is there a possibility of overeating?

To sum up, yes! You can also consume a lot of fat as well. Even though a Ketogenic diet will keep you full and naturally prevent yourself from overeating since you will be keeping your carb intake low. There's still the possibility of overeating, so make sure to stay alert.

How much a Ketogenic diet cost? Will it help to lost weight?

The amount of weight that you might lose completely depends on your body type and your physical activity. Adding exercise to your daily routine will accelerate the rate at which you lose weight. Cutting down various food procures such as sweeting agents, dairy products, wheat items will help.

As for the cost, it will also depend on you and your lifestyle. If you focus more on veggies to prepare your meal plan, then it might cost you a little less.

Won't eating so much fat hamper the heart health?
The primary fat groups that we generally consume are saturated fats, Monosaturared fats, polyunsaturated fats. Previously, people used to believe that saturated fats were horrible for the body, however, nowadays that conception is being altered.
Saturated fats have been seen to be terrible for our health as they consist of trans fat.
On the other hand, polyunsaturated fats found in fish are great as they improve your cholesterol levels.
As for monounsaturated fat, they are also great and help to maintain a healthy balance in our body and decrease cholesterol levels.

Will you feel bad during your early Keto days?
Since your body will be going through a large dietary change, some people often experience Keto Flu.
This is explained in details in Chapter 1.

Is Alcohol allowed on the diet?
Surprisingly, Alcohols are allowed on a Ketogenic Diet, but you should stay wary! There are hidden carbs in Alcohol and you don't want more of those unwanted carbs to slip into your body.
Beer, wine and other mixed drinks have carbohydrates in them, so going for liquor might be your best option. Even so, try to stay away from flavored liquors and as they could hold hidden carbs in them.

What to do if you feel constipated?
It's pretty common for individuals to experience uneven bowel movements during the early days. Below are some tips that will help you to mitigate your bowel problems.

- Consume plenty of water
- Consume 1 teaspoon of Coconut oil
- Stop eating nuts if you do
- Try coffee or tea
- Try eating flax seeds or chia seeds
- Consume more fibrous vegetables
- Take magnesium supplements

Chapter 7: Preparing your pantry

Once you have nailed down the basics of the Ketogenic Diet, the next step for you is to decide how you are going to prepare your pantry. Meaning, the dietary restrictions!

Good news for you is that the food items that you will need to avoid is not that difficult and you won't have to forgo of all of your favorite food items.

The main thing to remember is that you are to avoid all kinds of foods that are high in carb, such as chocolates, candy, sugary drinks, pasta, bread etc.

So, before going into the detailed list, you should eliminate any high carb food items from your pantry to prepare it for the days to come.

After that, star to restock your pantry following the below mentioned food guidelines.

Meats And Animal Produces: While choosing your meat, always make sure to avoid farmed animal meats and processed meats such as sausages or hot dogs. Try to go for the animal meats and animal derived products:

- Offal from grass-fed animals: kidney, liver, tripe, tongue etc
- Butter
- Gelatin
- Ghee
- Pastured eggs
- Pastured poultry and pork
- Seafood caught in the wild such as caviar, crab, mussels, clams and scallops
- Wild caught fish such as cod, mackerel, tuna, eel etc.
- Grass-fed meat such as lamb, venison, beef, lamb, chicken, rabbit etc.

Fats: Try to take more saturated and Monosaturared varieties of fat.

- Saturated fats include lard, tallow, duck fat, chicken fat, ghee etc.
- Monosaturared fats include avocado oil, olive oil and macadamia oil
- Fats rich in poly-saturated Omega-3s extracted from animal sources
- Cocoa butter, coconut butter
- 90% or higher dark chocolate
- Palm shortening
- Chia seeds

Vegetables: When choosing your vegetable, try to avoid root vegetables and stick to the green leafy ones as they will help you to keep your carbohydrates level at a minimum.

- Watercress
- Zucchini
- Spinach

- Tomatoes
- Shallots
- Seaweeds
- Pumpkin
- Scallions
- Radishes
- Okra
- Onions
- Mushrooms
- All leafy greens
- Lettuce
- Garlic
- Fennel
- Cucumber
- Chives
- Cauliflower
- Chives
- Celery
- Carrots
- Cabbage
- Broccoli
- Bell Pepper
- Asparagus
- Artichokes

Fruits: In terms of a Ketogenic diet, most fruits are off the table, mainly because of the high level of fructose. However, small amounts of berries are allowed.
Good choices for fruits are:

- Avocado
- Olives
- Blackberry
- Lime
- Lemon
- Blueberry
- Raspberry
- Strawberry
- Cranberry

Legumes: Similar to fruits, all types of legumes are off the table. However, very small amount of peas or green beans can be included in your diet.

Dairy Products: In general, the following dairy products are good for your soul

- Kefir
- Full fat yogurt
- Full fat raw cheese
- Full fat cottage cheese
- Heavy whipping cream
- Full fat sour cream
- Full fat cream cheese
- Ghee
- Butter

Drinks: All types of sweet or aerated drinks are to be avoided completely in your Keto diet. Drink of plenty of water though! Good drinks include:

- Coconut milk
- Almond milk
- Cashew milk
- Broth and soups
- Herbal teas
- Coffee teas
- Water
- Seltzer water
- Club soda
- Lemon and lime juices
- Sparkline water
- Water

Nuts and Seeds: In general nuts and seeds are allowed, but you should try to keep your intake at low levels since they enhance your carbohydrate intake. Be cautious while consuming nuts. However, keep In mind that you are to avoid peanuts as they fall under the legume category.
The following are allowed though:

- Almonds
- Macadamias
- Hazelnuts
- Pecans
- Pistachios
- Pine nuts
- Pumpkin seeds
- Sesame seeds
- Psyllium seeds
- Sunflower seeds
- Cashew nuts
- Walnuts

- Chia seeds

Herbs And Spices: As for herbs and spices, you are allowed to experiment with a wide variety of spices and herbs in order to enhance the flavor of your meals. Just make sure to avoid store-bough spices and herb that have hidden sugars of MSG's as they would be break your Keto diet.

Recommended spices include:

- Black pepper
- White pepper
- Sea salt
- Basil
- Chili powder
- Curry powder
- Italian seasoning
-
- Cumin powder
- Oregano
- Thyme
- Sage
- Rosemary
- Turmeric
- Parsley
- Cilantro
- Cinnamon
- Cloves
- Allspices
- Paprika
- Ginger
- Cardamom

Part 2: Time Saving Strategy

Chapter 8: Meal Prep And Amazing Time Saving Strategies

Given that you have gone through the previous pages, you should have a good grasp of the basics of Ketogenic Diet! So, we are now ready to move on to the Meal Prepping part of our book.

Throughout the following chapter, I will walk you through the basics of Meal Prepping and a number of awesome time saving techniques. Incorporating these techniques into your diet will further increase the efficiency of your Ketogenic Diet to a greater degree.

That being said, Meal Prepping is perhaps one of the most important and crucial aspect of any diet and this is the part that is ignored the most.

So, what exactly is Meal Prep?

In the strictest terms, the core objective of Meal Prepping is to provide you with a blueprint as to how you are going to make preparations for your diet.

However, if you are not following a diet, you can still create a rough meal plan about the foods that you are going to eat for the rest of the week!

In our case though, we are focusing on a Ketogenic Meal Plan!

However, dissecting the concept even further, we are able to get the definition below:

"Meal Prepping is the process of planning what you are going to eat (and how you are going to make it) ahead of time."

The advantages of Meal Prep

- It helps you to save a lot of money by allowing you to set up a rough estimate of your food budget ahead of time
- If allows you to stick to a healthy plan and eat as much healthy food as possible
- It minimizes food wastage
- It clears off the burden of "What you should cook next" and eases your mind, clearing it up of any food related stress.
- Prevent the wasting of time by letting you know exactly "What" you are going to eat and "When".

- Help you avoid monotony in your daily meal by spicing up the routine from time to time.
- Meal Prepping helps you to control your portions by adjusting a set amount of food per meal, this give you greater control over what you eat, helping in weight loss as well
- Greater control of your food routine will help you create a more balanced and nutritious diet plan in the long run
- Since everything is pre-planned, it will help you to avoid the rush of "Last minute preparations" and make the cooking process easier for you
- Meal Prepping will help you to seamlessly multi-task between other important works, as opposed to sitting in the kitchen all day to cook. Since you will keep everything prepared, it will save a lot of time from your daily routine and allow you to focus on other activities.

Amazing meal prep ideas

Keep in mind that there is a whole load of amazing Meal Prep ideas that you can find all around!

The following ideas are given to inspire you into coming up with your own ideas, and at the same time give you some pointers as to how you can start your journey.

Make a plant ahead of time: If you are reading this book, then you have probably decided to go on a Clean Eating diet journey. A good way to start this off is to start with a small number of recipes, for perhaps 7 days. Choose which recipes you are going to use and make a rough idea inside your head. Make a list and buy the ingredients accordingly ahead of time.

Keep a good supply of mason jars: Mason jars are terrific, not only for storing memories! But also for storing healthy salads! Assuming that you are a healthy buff, it might be a good idea to prepare your salads ahead of time and store them in mason jars. Make sure to keep the salad dressing at the bottom of the jar to ensure that nothing greens don't get soggy!

Three way seasoning in one pan: If your diet requires you to stick with lean meats such as chicken, then seasoning them from time to time might become somewhat of a chore. A simple solution to that is to prepare a pan with aluminum foil dividers. Using these will allow you to season three or more (depending on how many dividers you are using) types of chicken seasoning to be done using the same pan!

Boil eggs in an oven instead of a pot: Now this might sound a little bit weird at first, but it is high effective to say the least! The problem here comes with the quantity of eggs that can be boiled in one go. If you are using a standard sized pot, then you would probably be able to squeeze in 5 or 6 eggs max in one batch.

However, if you try to bake your eggs in muffin tins using an oven, then you will be able to get a dozen or perfectly hard-boiled eggs in no time!

Keep your prepared smoothies frozen in muffin tins: Plopping out a number of different ingredients early in the morning might be a chore for some people. A simple solution to that is to go ahead and freeze up your blended smoothies in muffin tins. This will not only save up time, but will also give you a delicious dose of satisfaction as you wake up in the morning and toss a few "smoothie cups" into the blender for a simple yet healthy breakfast.

Roast vegetables that require the same time in one batch: When you are preparing large batches of vegetables for roasting, it is smart to go ahead and create batches of vegetables depending on how long they take to roast. For example, you can create a batch of rapid cooking vegetables such as mushrooms, asparagus or cherry tomatoes and a batch of slow roasting vegies such as potatoes, cauliflowers and carrots in order to minimize time loss and maximize output.

Learn to effectively use a skewer: When you think of skewers, you automatically think of kabobs! But Skewers aren't necessarily designed to be used only with street meats. Wooden skewers can actually help you to measure how much meat you are going to consume in one go. So, you can punch in your meat in multiple skewers and divide them evenly and store them for the rest of the week. When the time comes, just take out one skewer and cook it up!

Keep a good supply of sectioned plastic containers: Sectioned containers like the one shown above are an absolute necessity for serious meal prepping savants! These will effortlessly give you enough space to separate each and every single component of your meal while making sure that you don't mix everything up and create a mess. The separate ingredients would also be really easy to find and use!

Keep a tab of your accomplishments: This is perhaps the most essential aspect of a Meal Prepping routine. Always make sure to somehow measure your progress and set small milestones for you to accomplish. Achieving these milestones will encourage you and inspire you further to keep pushing yourself until your reach your final goal. Alternatively, looking at your positive progress will greatly motivate you to push forward as well!

Why should you practice meal prepping on a Ketogenic diet?

If you are an extremely busy individual, then Meal Prepping will help you a lot during your Ketogenic Diet!

If you plan your meals ahead of time, it will help you to keep your mind free from the frustration of always thinking what you are going to eat next! And allow you to focus on your diet properly.

Having everything prepared beforehand will also make things easier for you and prevent you from slipping out of ketosis.
It will improve the effectiveness of your Ketogenic diet in the long term as well.

What to do with your leftovers?

Meal prepping always encourages storing and saving your leftovers for later using! Always make sure to store them in their appropriate containers and store in fridge for later use.

Tips to Prevent Cross-Contamination

During your Ketogenic Meal Prep journey, you will be dealing with both meat and vegetables, so it is highly advised that you follow the tips mentioned below in order to avoid the spreading of food-borne diseases.

- Always make sure to wash your hand thoroughly with warm water alongside your cutting boards, knives, counters and other utensils.
- Always make sure to use different bowls and dishes for different types of meats and vegetables.
- When storing the meat in fridge, make sure to keep the raw meat, seafood, poultry and eggs on the bottom shelf of your fridge and in individual sealed containers.
- Keep your refrigerator shelves cleaned and juices from meat/vegetables might drip on them.
- Always try to avoid keeping raw meat and vegetables and cooked meals together
- Always make sure to clean your cutting boards and use different cutting boards for different types of foods. Raw meats, vegetables and other foods should not be cut using the same table.

Early mistakes to avoid

Even though Meal Prepping is not that difficult to follow, there are some mistakes that you should avoid early on!
To ensure that you do not make the same mistakes, let me outline a few!

- Don't keep your food for too long out as they might very easily get contaminated with germs of bacteria,

- Don't rush when washing and rinsing your vegetables. Putting a little time there won't destroy your daily routine! Take your time and thoroughly wash your vegies before processing them.
- You should always make sure that you are heating your foods properly. Overheating them will burn them up while not heating them enough will leave harmful bacteria on the surface of the food. Use a meat thermometer if possible when dealing with meats.

Meal Prep FAQ's

If this if your first time, then it's almost certain that you are going to have some questions regarding Meal Prep.

Let me clear some of the most common one's for you before letting you go into the recipes!

Q1. How long does stored food usually last?

As a rule of thumb, you should not store your food for more than 4 days in air tight containers.

Q2. How should you store meal prepped food?

A good way is to use plastic containers to store the cooked food. Make sure to allow your meals to cool for 30-40 minutes before sealing them though.

Q3. What does buffet meal prep mean?

A buffet meal prep is when you batch cook a number of different ingredients and then create meals during the week as you keep on going, instead of prepping all the meals at once.

Q4. What type of containers should you use?

Plastic containers are BPA free, microwave and dishwasher safe so these are really cool to use.

Q5. How should you motivate yourself to meal prep every week?

Good pointers to remember is that meal prep will help you to stay healthy, energy and maintain a very healthy physique! And most importantly, it will help you save up a lot of money.

Q6. Is Freezing good?

While freezing meals are not recommended (as re-heating them sometimes diminishes the flavor), you are more than welcome to chill sauces, soups, chilis etc. and thaw them when needed.

Q7. How are you to re-heat workweek lunches without ruining them?

When you are in the office, re-heat your meals using the office microwave, and while at home...try to re-heat your meal in oven or stove (it preserves the flavor almost perfectly)

And that pretty much covers the basics of Meal Prep!

Now, let's dig deep into a step by step guide as to how you can actually prepare a healthy meal plan.

Chapter 9: Time Saving Kitchen Tools And Meal Prep Ideas

Meal Prepping requires a certain level of commitment to pull off! Starting with the basic preparations of your kitchen.

Preparing your kitchen

If you are new in this Meal Prepping though, the following are some of the essential tools that you should have in your kitchen!

Cutting Boards: Try to get boards that are made from solid materials such as plastic, glass, rubber or marble! These are mostly corrosion resistant and the non-porous surface makes it easier to clean them than wood.

Tools and Equipment: the most basic ones include

Measuring cups: Required to measure out spices and condiments.

Various sized spoons: The multiple sized spoons will allow you to measure out small amounts of spices.

Glass bowls and non-metallic containers: They are required for storing the meat alongside marinade.

Packaging materials (mentioned above): The materials are mentioned above and they can be used to store the meat in the fridge.

Kitchen and paper towels: These are required draining the meat.

Cold Storage Space (fridge will suffice): Since the meats are required to be kept under 40 degree Fahrenheit, a fridge should be enough.

Knives: Sharp knives should be used to slice the meat accordingly. While using the knife, you should keep the following in mind.

- Always make sure to use a sharp knife
- Never hold a knife under your arm or leave it under a piece of meat
- Always keep your knives within visible distance
- Always keep your knife point down
- Always cut down towards the cutting surface and away from your body
- Never allow children to toy with knives unattended
- Wash the knives while cutting different types of food

Mesh glove for protection: Cutting the meat requires precision as you will be using a very sharp knife. The following types of glove should be kept in mind:

- **Rubber gloves**
- **Butchering Gloves**
- **Mesh Glove**

Kitchen Scale for measurement: A kitchen scale will allow you to get accurate measurements of slightly pieces of meat and condiments.

Internal Thermometer: A meat thermometer will help you to measure the internal temperature of the jerky to ensure that you are able to ensure that the jerky are ready.

Baking Sheet: These are flat, rectangular metal pan that are used in oven, mainly for flat products such as sheet cakes, cookies etc.

Colander: A colander is a bowl-shaped kitchen utensil with holes that allows you to drain food such as pasta or rice. These are also use to rinsed veggies.

Aluminum Foil: Also known as misnomer tin foil, these are used to wrap up and cover food.

The importance of storage containers

Asides from the different the above mentioned instruments and appliances, another core aspect of Meal Prepping are "Containers".

In fact, storage containers are the beating heart of a Meal Prepping program as you have to store a lot of your left-overs for later consumption.

However, purchasing a good storage container isn't as easy as it sounds! Mainly because of the sheer amount of variety available in the market.

That being said though, the following information should help you make the right decision for you meal.

The two main type of containers that you should know about are Glass containers and Plastic containers. (A third option, "Stainless Steel" containers are briefly discussed shortly as well)

To make the decision easier for you, the core difference between the wo types of containers are as follows:

Facts about Glass Containers

- Glass containers are a bit more expensive but are ideal for long term storage
- Due to their heavy weight, glass containers are not ideal for "on-the-go" eating
- They are easier to clean
- If you are concerned about plastic safety, then these are the ones to go with!

Facts about Plastic Containers

- Easy to carry and lightweight, ideal for individuals who are always on the go
- They are more convenience and come in a wide variety of sizes and shapes

- They are easy to dispose

Now that you are familiar with the core differences between the two, let me focus on some of the key components that you should keep an eye out for while buying your new and fancy container!

- Always make sure to go for containers that are leak proof and have a tight lid. Some containers come with "Snap-On" lids! However, if you are on a tighter budget, you can go for normal containers as well from good brands such as Glad or Rubbermaid.
- Always make sure to go for containers that are clearly labeled "Microwave Safe". Asides from the fact that normal containers will instantly melt in your Microwave, they will also hamper the texture and flavor of your meal and make it unappealing in the long run. However, if you want to avoid risk of plastic flavor altogether, go for glass containers!
- If you plan on freezing your goods for long time, then it is highly advised that you buy containers that are specially designed to sustain extreme temperatures. Even though freezing is amazing for long term storage, if you don't store them properly, your foods might suffer from "Freezer Burn" (Generally causes white patches on food that hampers flavor). Thick glassed mason jars and Freezer specific Ziploc bags are excellent for long term Freezer storage.
- Stainless Steel containers are excellent for preventing Freeze burns as well and are great for container smoothie type foods or meals that have meat in them.

Some good containers that you should consider are:

- Glasslock 18 piece Assorted Oven-Safe Container (45$)
- LunchBots Trio Stainless Steel Food Container (25$)
- Snapware Total Solution Pyrex Glass Food Storage 10-Piece Set (23$)
- ReCap Mason Jars (15$)
- Stashers Reusable Silicone Food Bags (12$)
- Anchor Hocking 4 Cup Round Food Storage Container (4$)
- Rubbermaid Plastic Containers – Set of 42 (20$)
- MealPrep's Premium Glass Containers- set of 6 (18.99$)

A Note On BPA

When consider plastic containers, some people often think about the risk that relating to "BPA".

For those of you who are not familiar with BPA, it is a kind of chemical substance that is used to make plastic clear and hard. These are also used to manufacture re-usable water bottles, baby bottles etc.

However, it is largely believed that this is a chemical that is toxic to the human body and may cause health issues.
This is a good concern, but you should know that high quality food containers are very thoroughly checked and follow FDA regulations to ensure that the BPA levels are at the base minimum level.
So, as long as you are going with good quality containers, there should be no issue.

Chapter 10: 3 Weeks Meal Plan

With that you should have a good idea about the basics of Meal Planning. Now, let me walk you through the core concepts as to how you can "Actually" prepare for your Meal Prepping journey.

The core steps of Meal Prep

There is a very close relation between Meal Plan and Meal Prepping and some people often tend to mix the two together!
Meal Planning is creating an outline of what you are going to eat. On the other hand, Meal Planning is how you are going to prepare your ingredients in order to follow the said meal plan.
That being said, this chapter will provide you with a simple Keto Meal Plan while giving you some pointers on how you can create your own personalized meal plan.
That being said, there are essentially four steps to creating a meal plan. The steps below are illustrated by keeping a sample meal plan in mind.

Step 1: Choosing a Day

The first step into creating your meal prep guide is to choose the days when you will prepare your ingredients.
Weekends are amazing for this job as you will be able to get the most out of your day. Not to mention the fact that you will be able to get the help of your family members as well.
When beginning though, you should not plan meals for the whole week as it might be too much! Try to prepare three meals at the beginning and keep increasing the number as you become more proficient.

Step 2: Choose your meals

Once you have chosen the meal prepping days, next choose the meals that you are going to prepare for breakfast, lunch and dinner.
When choosing the recipes, make sure to maintain the macronutrient goals based on your dietary requirements.

Step 3: Equipment and Shopping List

Assuming that we have the following ingredients

- 2.5 pound of chicken meat
- 2 large bags of mixed vegetables such as broccoli, carrots, cauliflower etc.
- 2 and a ½ pound of sweet potatoes
- Salt and pepper as needed alongside any seasoning mix that you might need

As for the equipment

- 2 baking sheets
- Aluminum foil as needed
- A large sized pot
- Colander
- Cutting board
- Knife
- Non-stick cooking spray
- Containers such as plastic containers or bags

Keep in mind that all of the equipment have already been discussed in the previous chapter.

Step 4: The Process

Keep in mind that the meal prepping process will vary from one meal to the next, the following is simply for the ingredient list provided above.

- Take a large sized pot and dump the vegetables, add water until the veggies are covered and boil the vegetables properly
- While you are boiling your vegetables, pre-heat your oven to 350 degree Fahrenheit
- Take the baking sheet and cover with aluminum foil, spray with non-stick cooking spray. Transfer the chicken thigh and season with salt and pepper as needed
- Bake them for 25 minutes
- While baking, Wash the potatoes well and cut them very carefully into rounds and slice the rounds into smaller chunks
- Transfer the chunks to another baking sheet and transfer the sheet to your oven, bake for 30 minutes

- By now the veggies should be ready, so take them out and strain them in a colander
- Take five different plastic containers and add the veggies to the container
- If you want, then you may portion them out as needed
- The chicken should be ready now, so take them out and portion them between the containers
- Do the same for the sweet potatoes

And that's about it!
Follow a template such as this when creating your very own meal plans.

A Sample 21 Days Meal Plan

<u>Week 1</u>

Week 1	Breakfast	Lunch	Dinner
Day 1 (Sunday)	Meal Prep Day	Meal Prep Day	Meal Prep Day
Day 2 (Monday)	The Greek Cucumber Salad	Delicious Broccoli Tilapia	Fantastic Garlic And Butter Cod
Day 3 (Tuesday)	Simple Cobb Salad	Fantastic Asian Beef Steak	Simple Parmesan Baked Chicken
Day 4 (Wednesday)	The Greek Cucumber Salad	Delicious Broccoli Tilapia	Fantastic Garlic And Butter Cod
Day 5 (Thursday)	Simple Cobb Salad	Fantastic Asian Beef Steak	Simple Parmesan Baked Chicken
Day 6 (Friday)	The Greek Cucumber Salad	Delicious Broccoli Tilapia	Fantastic Garlic And Butter Cod
Day 7 (Saturday)	Meal Prep Day	Meal Prep Day	Meal Prep Day

<u>Reference for Week 1 Shopping List</u>
For Breakfast

Recipe 1: The Greek Cucumber Salad

- ½ cup olive oil
- 2 tablespoons red wine vinegar
- 1 teaspoon dried oregano
- 1 teaspoon garlic salt
- Pinch of salt
- Pinch of ground black pepper
- 4 cucumbers, peeled and sliced into rounds, then quartered

- 4 tomatoes, diced
- 1 red onion, thinly sliced
- 2 cups black olives, pitted and sliced
- 1 cup feta cheese, crumbled
- 2 cups sliced pepperoni slices, halved

Recipe 2: Simple Cobb Salad

- 4 cups romaine lettuce, chopped
- 6 perfectly cooked bacon, crumbled
- 4 hardboiled eggs, peeled and sliced
- 2 cups ham, cubed
- 1 cup crumbled blue cheese
- 2 avocados, sliced
- 1 cup cherry tomatoes, sliced
- 3 scallions, white green parts chopped
- Dairy free Ranch dressing

For Lunch

Recipe 1: Delicious Broccoli Tilapia

- 6 ounce of tilapia, frozen
- 1 tablespoon of butter
- 1 tablespoon of garlic, minced
- 1 teaspoon of lemon pepper seasoning
- 1 cup of broccoli florets, fresh

Recipe 2: Fantastic Asian Beef Steak

- 2 tablespoon of sriracha sauce
- 1 tablespoon of garlic, minced
- 1 tablespoon of ginger, freshly grated
- 1 yellow bell pepper, cut in strips
- 1 red bell pepper cut in thin strips
- 1 tablespoon of sesame oil, garlic flavored
- 1 tablespoon of stevia
- ½ a teaspoon of curry powder
- ½ a teaspoon of rice wine vinegar
- 8 ounce of beef sirloin cut into strips
- 2 cups of baby spinach, stemmed
- ½ head of butter of lettuce, torn

For Dinner

Recipe 1: Fantastic Garlic And Butter Cod

- 3 cod fillets, 8 ounces each
- ¾ pound baby bok choy, halved
- 1/3 cup butter, thinly sliced
- 1 and ½ tablespoons garlic, minced
- Salt and pepper to taste

Recipe 2: Simple Parmesan Baked Chicken

- 2 tablespoons ghee
- 2 boneless chicken breasts, skinless
- Pink salt
- Freshly ground black pepper
- ½ cup mayonnaise
- ¼ cup parmesan cheese, grated
- 1 tablespoon dried Italian seasoning
- ¼ cup crushed pork rinds

<u>**Week 2**</u>

Week 2	Breakfast	Lunch	Dinner
Day 1 (Sunday)	Meal Prep Day	Meal Prep Day	Meal Prep Day
Day 2 (Monday)	Satisfying Berry Smoothie	Garlic And Parsley Chicken Feast	Magical Cucumber Soup
Day 3 (Tuesday)	Kale And Avocado In A Skillet	Cool Balsamic Chicken And Veggies	Delightful Spring Salad
Day 4 (Wednesday)	Satisfying Berry Smoothie	Garlic And Parsley Chicken Feast	Magical Cucumber Soup
Day 5 (Thursday)	Kale And Avocado In A Skillet	Cool Balsamic Chicken And Veggies	Delightful Spring Salad
Day 6 (Friday)	Satisfying Berry Smoothie	Garlic And Parsley Chicken Feast	Magical Cucumber Soup
Day 7 (Saturday)	Meal Prep Day	Meal Prep Day	Meal Prep Day

<u>**Reference for Week 2 Shopping List**</u>
For Breakfast
Recipe 1: Satisfying Berry Smoothie

- ¼ cup frozen blueberries
- ¼ cup frozen blackberries
- 1 cup unsweetened almond milk
- 1 teaspoon vanilla bean extract
- 3 teaspoons flaxseed
- 1 scoop chilled Greek yogurt
- Stevia as needed

Recipe 2: Kale And Avocados In A Skillet

- 2 tablespoons olive oil, divided
- 2 cups mushrooms, sliced
- 5 ounces fresh kale, stemmed and sliced into ribbons
- 1 avocado, sliced
- 4 large eggs
- Salt and pepper as needed

For Lunch

Recipe 1: Garlic And Parsley Chicken Feast

- 1 tablespoon dry parsley
- 1 tablespoon dry basil
- 4 chicken breast halves, boneless and skinless
- ½ teaspoon salt
- ½ teaspoon red pepper flakes, crushed
- 2 tomatoes, sliced

Recipe 2: Cool Balsamic Chicken And Veggies

- 8 chickne thigh, boneless and skinless
- 10 stalks asparagus, halved
- 2 peppers, cut in chunks
- 1 red onion, diced
- ½ cup carrots, sliced
- 2 garlic cloves, minced
- 5 ounces mushrooms, diced
- ¼ cup baslamic vinegar
- 2 tablespoons olive oil
- ½ teaspoon stevia
- ½ tablespoon oregano
- Salt and pepper to taste

For Dinner

Recipe 1: Magical Cucumber Soup

- 2 tablespoons garlic, minced
- 4 cups english cucumbers, peeled and diced
- ½ cup onions, diced
- 1 tablespoon lemon juice
- 1 and ½ cups vegetable broth
- ½ teaspoon salt
- ¼ teaspoon red pepper flakes
- ¼ cup parsley, diced
- ½ cup Greek yogurt, plain

Recipe 2: Delightful Spring Salad

- 2 ounces mixed green vegetables
- 3 tablespoons roasted pine nuts
- 2 tablespoons 5 minutes 5 Keto Raspberry Vinaigrete
- 2 tablespoons Shaved Parmesan
- Salt and pepper to taste

Week 3	Breakfast	Lunch	Dinner
Day 1 (Sunday)	Meal Prep Day	Meal Prep Day	Meal Prep Day
Day 2 (Monday)	Smoked Salmon And Cream Cheese Rolls	Generous Tomato And Basil Soup	Roasted Brussels And Parmesan
Day 3 (Tuesday)	Heart Throb Denver Omelette	Juicy Steak And Broccoli Delight	Garlic And Parsley Chicken Feast
Day 4 (Wednesday)	Smoked Salmon And Cream Cheese Rolls	Generous Tomato And Basil Soup	Roasted Brussels And Parmesan
Day 5 (Thursday)	Heart Throb Denver Omelette	Juicy Steak And Broccoli Delight	Garlic And Parsley Chicken Feast
Day 6 (Friday)	Smoked Salmon And Cream Cheese Rolls	Generous Tomato And Basil Soup	Roasted Brussels And Parmesan
Day 7 (Saturday)	Meal Prep Day	Meal Prep Day	Meal Prep Day

Reference for Week 3 Shopping List
For Breakfast

Recipe 1: Smoked Salmon And Cream Cheese Rolls

- 4 ounces cream cheese, at room temperature
- 1 teaspoon grated lemon zest
- 1 teaspoon Dijon mustard
- 2 tablespoons scallions, chopped (white and green parts)
- Pink salt
- Freshly ground black pepper
- 1 pack (4 ounces) cold-smoked salmon (12 slices)

Recipe 2: Heart Throb Denver Omelette

- 2 tablespoons butter
- ¼ cup onion, chopped
- ¼ cup green bell pepper, diced
- ¼ cup grape tomatoes, halved
- 2 whole eggs
- ¼ cup ham, chopped

For Lunch

Recipe 1: Generous Tomato And Basil Soup

- 2 tablespoons olive oil
- 1 yellow onion, diced
- 2 garlic cloves, minced
- 2 cans (28 ounces) whole peeled tomatoes, with juice
- 2 cups vegetable broth
- ½ cup salted butter
- ½ cup basil leaves, chopped
- 1 cup heavy whipping cream
- Salt and pepper as needed

Recipe 2: Juicy Steak And Broccoli Delight

- 4 ounces butter
- ¾ pound Ribeye steak, sliced
- 9 ounces broccoli, chopped
- 1 yellow onion, sliced
- 1 tablespoon coconut aminos
- 1 tablespoon pumpkin seeds
- Salt and pepper to taste

For Dinner

Recipe 1: Roasted Brussels And Parmesan

- 1 pound brusels sprouts
- 1 tablespoon olive oil
- Salt and pepper
- ¼ cup parmesan cheese, either shaved or grated
- ¼ cup whole, skinless hazelnuts

Recipe 2: Garlic And Parsley Chicken Feast

- 1 tablespoon dry parsley
- 1 tablespoon dry basil
- 4 chicken breast halves, boneless and skinless
- ½ teaspoon salt
- ½ teaspoon red pepper flakes, crushed
- 2 tomatoes, sliced

Part 3: Quick And Easy Keto Recipes

Chapter 11: Starters And Snacks

Mozzarella Bacon Crunchies
Serving: 4
Prep Time: 10 minutes
Cook Time: 5 minutes
Ingredients

- 8 bacon strips
- 4 mozarella string cheese pieces
- Olive oil, as needed

How To

1. Take a heavy duty skillet and place it over medium heat
2. Add 2 inch of oil, let it heat up to 350 degree F (check using thermometer)
3. Cut the string cheese to 8 pieces
4. Wrap each piece string cheese with a strip of bacon and secure using toothpick
5. Cook the sticks in hot oil for 2 minutes until the bacons are browned
6. Transfer to serving platter and drain with kitchen towel
7. Serve!

Nutrition (Per Serving)

- Calories: 278
- Fat: 15g
- Carbohydrates: 3g
- Protein: 32g

Storage Options/Meal Prep Tips: Transfer to airtight containers and serve when needed, possible to refrigerate for 3 days. Freezer time 3-4 months.

Awesome Berry-Avocado Smoothie

Serving: 2
Prep Time: 5 minutes
Cook Time: Nil
<u>Ingredients</u>

- 1 cup unsweetened full-fat coconut milk
- 1 scoop Perfect Keto Exogenous Ketone Powder in peaches and cream
- ½ avocado
- 1 cup fresh spinach
- ½ cup berries, fresh or frozen
- ½ cup ice cubes
- ¼ teaspoon liquid stevia

<u>How To</u>

1. Add the listed ingredients to a blender
2. Blend well until properly mixed and frothy
3. Pour into tall glass
4. Enjoy!

<u>Nutrition (Per Serving)</u>

- Calories: 355
- Fat: 40g
- Carbohydrates: 8g
- Protein: 4g

Storage Options/Meal Prep Tips: Transfer to mason jars and store in your fridge for 3-4 days.

Blistered Green Beans And Almond Delight

Serving: 4
Prep Time: 10 minutes
Cook Time: 20 minutes
<u>**Ingredients**</u>

- 1 pound fresh green beans, ends trimmed
- 1 and ½ tablespoons olive oil
- ¼ teaspoon salt
- 1 and ½ tablespoons fresh dill, minced
- Juice of one lemon
- ¼ cup crushed almonds
- Flaky salt

<u>How To</u>

1. Pre-heat your oven to 400 degree F
2. Add the green beans to a bowl and toss with olive oil and salt
3. Spread the blistered beans in a single layer on a large sized sheet pan
4. Roast for 10 minutes and give it a nice stir, roast for 8 minutes more
5. Remove from the oven and keep stirring while adding the lemon juice and dill
6. Top with crushed almonds and flake salt
7. Serve!

<u>Nutrition (Per Serving)</u>

- Calories: 347
- Fat: 16g
- Carbohydrates: 5g
- Protein: 45g

Storage Options/Meal Prep Tips: Transfer to airtight containers and serve when needed, possible to refrigerate for 3 days. Freezer time 3-4 months.

Cheesy Tuna Bites

Serving: 2
Prep Time: 10 minutes
Cook Time: 10 minutes
<u>Ingredients</u>

- 10 ounces Canned Tuna, drained
- ¼ cup Keto Friendly mayonnaise
- 1 medium avocado, cubed
- ¼ cup parmesan cheese
- 1/3 cup almond flour
- ½ teaspoon garlic powder
- ¼ teaspoon onion powder
- Salt and pepper as needed
- ½ cup coconut oil

<u>How To</u>

1. Take a mixing bowl and add the listed ingredients except coconut oil and avocado
2. Take the cubed avocado and carefully fold them in the tuna mix
3. Mix well and turn the mixture into balls
4. Roll the balls into almond flour
5. Take a pan over medium heat and add coconut oil
6. Allow the oil to heat up
7. Add tuna balls and cook them well until you have a brown texture
8. Serve and enjoy!

<u>Nutrition (Per Serving)</u>

- Calories: 134
- Fat: 11g
- Carbohydrates: 2g
- Protein: 7g

Storage Options/Meal Prep Tips: Transfer to airtight containers and serve when needed, possible to refrigerate for 3 days. Freezer time 3-4 months.

Caramelized Cool Endives

Serving: 4
Prep Time: 5 minutes
Cook Time: 10 minutes
Ingredients

- 2 pounds endive
- 4 and ¼ ounces butter
- ½ teaspoon salt
- ¼ teaspoon pepper
- 1 tablespoon fresh chives, chopped

How To

1. Cut endives into inch sized pieces
2. Take a large frying pan and place it over high heat
3. Add butter and melt
4. Add endive to the pan and stir cook until slightly browned
5. Lower heat to low and keep stirring until the liquid has evaporated and endives are caramelized
6. Season with salt and pepper
7. Serve with a garnish of chopped parsley and chives
8. Enjoy!

Nutrition (Per Serving)

- Calories: 92
- Fat: 7g
- Carbohydrates: 8g
- Protein: 1g

Storage Options/Meal Prep Tips: Transfer to airtight containers and serve when needed, possible to refrigerate for 3 days. Freezer time 3-4 months.

Crunchy Pork Rinds And Zucchini Sticks

Serving: 2
Prep Time: 5 minutes
Cook Time: 25 minutes
<u>Ingredients</u>

- 2 medium zucchinis, halved lenghtwise and seeded
- ¼ cup crushed pork rinds
- ¼ cup grated parmesan cheese
- 2 garlic cloves, minced
- 2 tablespoons melted butter
- Salt and pepper
- Olive oil for drizzle

<u>How To</u>

1. Pre-heat your oven to 400 degree F
2. Line a baking sheet with aluminum foil
3. Place zucchini halves (cut side facing up) on prepared baking sheet
4. Take a medium bowl and add pork rinds, parmesan cheese, garlic, melted butter, season with pepper and salt
5. Mix well
6. Spoon pork rind mix onto zucchini stick
7. Drizzle olive oil
8. Bake for 20 minutes until the topping is golden brown
9. Turn your broiler and brown for 3-5 minutes
10. Serve and enjoy!

<u>Nutrition (Per Serving)</u>

- Calories: 231
- Fat: 20g
- Carbohydrates: 6g
- Protein: 9g

Storage Options/Meal Prep Tips: Transfer to airtight containers and serve when needed, possible to refrigerate for 4-6 days. Freezer time 3-4 month.

Crunchy Sprouts Chips

Serving: 4
Prep Time: 10 minutes
Cook Time: 10-15 minutes
<u>Ingredients</u>

- 1 pound brussels, washed and dried
- 2 tablespoons extra virgin olive oil
- 1 teaspoon kosher salt

<u>How To</u>

1. Pre-heat your oven to 400 degree F
2. Prepare the sprouts by trimming the stock and peels
3. Discard the outer leaves one by one all the way to the core
4. Transfer the leaves to a bowl
5. Add oil to the leaves and toss them well to coat them
6. Rub all over
7. Season with salt and pepper
8. Spread them evenly on baking sheet, making sure to spread the leaves apart as to prevent stacking
9. Bake for 10-15 minutes until deep brown
10. Remove from oven and allow them to cool
11. Sprinkle a bit of salt and serve

<u>Nutrition (Per Serving)</u>

- Calories: 104
- Fat: 7g
- Carbohydrates: 5g
- Protein: 3g

Storage Options/Meal Prep Tips: Transfer to airtight containers and serve when needed, possible to refrigerate for 3 days. Freezer time 3-4 months.

Heavy Chipotle Kale Chips

Serving: 4
Prep Time: 4 minutes
Cook Time: 29 minutes
<u>**Ingredients**</u>

- 2 large bunch kale, chopped into 4 pieces and stemmed
- 1 tablespoon olive oil
- 1/8 teaspoon salt
- 1 teaspoon chipotle powder
- ¼ cup parmesan cheese, shredded

<u>**How To**</u>

1. Wash kale thoroughly and dry, cut into 4 inch pieces
2. Pre-heat your oven to 250 degree F
3. Take a baking sheet and line with parchment paper
4. Take a bowl and add kale, coat the kale with olive oil, chipotle and cheese
5. Transfer the mix to baking sheet
6. Bake for 19 minutes and check the crispiness
7. If you need more crispiness, bake for 9 minutes more
8. Serve and enjoy!

<u>**Nutrition (Per Serving)**</u>

- Calories: 37
- Fat: 3g
- Carbohydrates: 3g
- Protein: 1g

Storage Options/Meal Prep Tips: Transfer to airtight containers and serve when needed, possible to refrigerate for 7 days.

Parmesan Rind And Green Beans

Serving: 2
Prep Time: 5 minutes
Cook Time: 15 minutes
<u>**Ingredients**</u>

- ½ pond fresh green beans
- 2 tablespoons crushed pork rinds
- 2 tablespoons olive oil
- 1 tablespoon Parmesan chees,e grated
- Salt and pepper as needed

<u>**How To**</u>

1. Pre-heat your oven to 400 degree F
2. Take a medium bowl and add green beans, pork rinds, olive oil, Parmesan
3. Season with pink salt, pepper and toss until beans are coated
4. Spread bean mix on baking sheet
5. Roast for 15 minutes, making sure to give it a shake at halfway point
6. Divide beans between two platters and serve
7. Enjoy!

<u>**Nutrition (Per Serving)**</u>

- Calories: 175
- Fat: 15g
- Carbohydrates: 5g
- Protein: 6g

Storage Options/Meal Prep Tips: Transfer to airtight containers and serve when needed, possible to refrigerate for 3 days. Freezer time 3-4 months.

Fantastic Zucchini Fries

Serving: 4
Prep Time: 5 minutes
Cook Time: 20 minutes
<u>Ingredients</u>

- 2 pounds zucchini
- 1 cup almond flour
- 1 cup parmesan cheese, grated
- 1 teaspoon onion powder
- ½ teaspoon black pepper
- 2 whole eggs
- 3 tablespoons olive oil

Tomato Mayo

- 1 cup Keto-Friendly Mayonnaise
- 1 teaspoon tomato paste
- ½ teaspoon cayenne pepper
- ½ teaspoon cayenne pepper
- Salt and pepper

<u>How To</u>

1. Add the mayo ingredients to a bowl and mix well
2. Pre-heat your oven to 400 degree F
3. Line up a baking sheet with parchment paper
4. Crack an egg into a shallow bowl and whisk until smooth
5. Add almond flour, parmesan cheese, spices in another bowl
6. Cut up the zucchini into sticks and remove the seeds
7. Dredge the zucchini into almond flour mix and cover it well
8. Dip them in the egg batter and again in the flour mix
9. Transfer the zucchini to baking sheet and drizzle olive oil
10. Bake for 20-25 minutes until the fries are browned
11. Serve with the mayo and enjoy!

<u>Nutrition (Per Serving)</u>

- Calories: 123
- Fat: 8g
- Carbohydrates: 12g
- Protein: 3g

Storage Options/Meal Prep Tips: Transfer to airtight containers and serve when needed, possible to refrigerate for 3 days. Freezer time 3-4 months.

Chapter 12: Salads

The Greek Cucumber Salad

Serving: 6
Prep Time: 15 minutes
Cook Time: Nil
Ingredients

- ½ cup olive oil
- 2 tablespoons red wine vinegar
- 1 teaspoon dried oregano
- 1 teaspoon garlic salt
- Pinch of salt
- Pinch of ground black pepper
- 4 cucumbers, peeled and sliced into rounds, then quartered
- 4 tomatoes, diced
- 1 red onion, thinly sliced
- 2 cups black olives, pitted and sliced
- 1 cup feta cheese, crumbled
- 2 cups sliced pepperoni slices, halved

How To

1. Take a small bowl and whisk in olive oil, vinegar, garlic salt, oregano, pepper and salt
2. Take a large bowl and add cucumbers, tomatoes, olives, onion, cheese and pepperoni
3. Pour dressing over top and toss until coated. Serve immediately and enjoy!

Nutrition (Per Serving)

- Calories: 590
- Fat: 55g
- Carbohydrates: 10g
- Protein: 12g

Storage Options/Meal Prep Tips: Prepare the ingredients and dressing beforehand. Store them in different zip bags and store in fridge for 2-3 days.

Caprese Avocado Salad

Serving: 6
Prep Time: 15 minutes
Cook Time: Nil
<u>Ingredients</u>

- 2 avocados, cubed
- 1 cup cherry tomatoes, halved
- 8 ounces mozzarella balls, halved
- 2 tablespoons finely chopped fresh basil
- 2 tablespoons olive oil
- 2 tablespoons balsamic vinegar
- 1 tablespoon salt
- Fresh ground black pepper

<u>How To</u>

1. Take a salad bowl and toss all the ingredients together and well mixed
2. Season with pepper
3. Serve immediately and enjoy!

<u>Nutrition (Per Serving)</u>

- Calories: 358
- Fat: 30g
- Carbohydrates: 9g
- Protein: 14g

Storage Options/Meal Prep Tips: Prepare the ingredients and dressing beforehand. Store them in different zip bags and store in fridge for 2-3 days.

Simple Cobb Salad

Serving: 6
Prep Time: 10 minutes
Cook Time: Nil
<u>Ingredients</u>

- 4 cups romaine lettuce, chopped
- 6 perfectly cooked bacon, crumbled
- 4 hardboiled eggs, peeled and sliced
- 2 cups ham, cubed
- 1 cup crumbled blue cheese
- 2 avocados, sliced
- 1 cup cherry tomatoes, sliced
- 3 scallions, white green parts chopped
- Dairy free Ranch dressing

<u>How To</u>

1. Divide the lettuce evenly amongst 4 large salad bowls
2. Top each with bacon, eggs, ham, cheese, avocados, tomatoes and scallions
3. Arrange the ingredients nicely
4. Top with your desired dressing
5. Serve immediately and enjoy!

<u>Nutrition (Per Serving)</u>

- Calories: 529
- Fat: 38g
- Carbohydrates: 5g
- Protein: 36g

Storage Options/Meal Prep Tips: Prepare the ingredients and dressing beforehand. Store them in different zip bags and store in fridge for 2-3

The Bacon And Blue cheese Kale Salad

Serving: 2
Prep Time: 10 minutes
Cook Time: 10 minutes
<u>**Ingredients**</u>

- 4 bacon slices
- 2 cups stemmed, chopped fresh kale
- 1 tablespoons vinaigrette Salad Dressing (check for Keto friendliness)
- Salt and pepper as needed
- ¼ cup pecans
- ¼ cup blue cheese crumbles

<u>**How To**</u>

1. Take a medium skillet and place it over medium-high heat
2. Cook the bacon for 8 minutes (both sides) until crispy
3. Transfer to paper towel-lined plate
4. Take a large bowl and massage kale with vinaigrette for 2 minutes
5. Add salt and pepper
6. Let it sit while the bacon cooks
7. Chop cooked bacon and pecans and add them to the bowl with kale
8. Toss well and sprinkle blue cheese
9. Toss again and portion onto two plates
10. Serve and enjoy!

<u>**Nutrition (Per Serving)**</u>

- Calories: 353
- Fat: 29g
- Carbohydrates: 7g
- Protein: 16g

Storage Options/Meal Prep Tips: Prepare the ingredients and dressing beforehand. Store them in different zip bags and store in fridge for 2-3

Amazing Chicken Caesar Salad

Serving: 4
Prep Time: 10 minutes
Cook Time: Nil
<u>**Ingredients**</u>

- 1 head romaine lettuce, chopped
- 4 (4 ounces) boneless, skinless chicken breast, cooked and cubed
- ½ cup Caesar dressing
- ½ cup grated parmesan cheese, divided

<u>**How To**</u>

1. Take a large bowl and toss lettuce, chicken and dressing alongside ¼ cup of Parmesan cheese
2. Add your desired toppings and serve with remaining ¼ cup of parmesan cheese sprinkled on top
3. Enjoy!

<u>**Nutrition (Per Serving)**</u>

- Calories: 343
- Fat: 20g
- Carbohydrates: 4g
- Protein: 33g

Storage Options/Meal Prep Tips: Prepare the ingredients and dressing beforehand. Store them in different zip bags and store in fridge for 2-

Hearty Shrimp And Arugula Salad

Serving: 8
Prep Time: 10 minutes
Cook Time: Nil
<u>Ingredients</u>

- 16 cups arugula
- 2 pounds shirmp, cooked and peeled
- 2 avocados, diced
- 8 tablespoons olive oil
- 4 lemon, 2 juiced and 2 cut in wedges
- Salt and pepper to taste

<u>How To</u>

1. Take a large bowl and add arugula, shrimp, avocado and mix
2. Add olive oil, salt, lemon juice and pepper
3. Mix well and serve with lemon wedges
4. Enjoy!

<u>Nutrition (Per Serving)</u>

- Calories: 328
- Fat: 24g
- Carbohydrates: 4g
- Protein: 6g

Storage Options/Meal Prep Tips: Store in airtight containers and refrigerate for up to 3 days until served!

Amazing Chopped Greek Salad

Serving: 2
Prep Time: 10 minutes
Cook Time: Nil
Ingredients

- 2 cups romaine, chopped
- ½ cup grape tomatoes
- ¼ cup sliced black olives, Kalamata
- ¼ cup feta cheese, crumbled
- 2 tablespoons Vinagrette Salad dressing
- Salt and pepper
- 1 tablespoon olive oil

How To

1. Take a large bowl and add romaine, tomatoes, vinaigrette, feta cheese and mix
2. Season with salt and pepper
3. Drizzle olive oil and toss
4. Divide the salad between bowls
5. Serve and enjoy!

Nutrition (Per Serving)

- Calories: 202
- Fat: 19g
- Carbohydrates: 3g
- Protein: 4g

Storage Options/Meal Prep Tips: Prepare the ingredients and dressing beforehand. Store them in different zip bags and store in fridge for 2-3

Delightful Spring Salad

Serving: 2
Prep Time: 10 minutes
Cook Time: 2 minutes
<u>**Ingredients**</u>

- 2 ounces mixed green vegetables
- 3 tablespoons roasted pine nuts
- 2 tablespoons 5 minutes 5 Keto Raspberry Vinaigrete
- 2 tablespoons Shaved Parmesan
- Salt and pepper to taste

<u>**How To**</u>

1. Cook the bacon until crispy
2. Take a bowl and add salad ingredients and crumble the crispy bacon into the salad
3. Mix well
4. Dress with your desired dressing
5. Serve and enjoy!

<u>**Nutrition (Per Serving)**</u>

- Calories: 209
- Fat: 17g
- Carbohydrates: 10g
- Protein: 4g

Storage Options/Meal Prep Tips: Store in airtight containers and refrigerate for up to 3 days until served!

Roasted Brussels With Parmesan

Serving: 2
Prep Time: 10 minutes
Cook Time: 15 minutes

<u>**Ingredients**</u>

- 1 pound brusels sprouts
- 1 tablespoon olive oil
- Salt and pepper
- ¼ cup parmesan cheese, either shaved or grated
- ¼ cup whole, skinless hazelnuts

<u>**How To**</u>

1. Pre-heat your oven to 350 degree F
2. Line baking sheet with silicone baking mat
3. Trim bottom and core the Brussels sprouts with a small knife
4. Put leaves in medium bowl
5. Toss leaves with olive oil and season with salt and pepper
6. Spread leaves in single layer on baking sheet and roast for 10-15 minutes
7. Divide Brussels sprouts leaves between two bowls
8. Top with shaved parmesan and hazelnuts
9. Serve and enjoy!

<u>**Nutrition (Per Serving)**</u>

- Calories: 267
- Fat: 19g
- Carbohydrates: 13g
- Protein: 14g

Storage Options/Meal Prep Tips: Prepare the ingredients and dressing beforehand. Store them in different zip bags and store in fridge for 2-3

Bacon, Avocado And Goat Cheese Salad

Serving: 2
Prep Time: 10 minutes
Cook Time: 20 minutes
Ingredients

- 8 oounces goat cheese
- 8 ounces bacon
- 2 whole avocados
- 4 ounces walnuts
- 4 ounces arugula lettuce

Dressing

- ½ a lemon, juiced
- ½ a cup Keto-Friendly mayonnaise
- ½ cup olive oil
- 2 tablespoons heavy whip cream

How To

1. Pre-heat your oven to 400 degree F
2. Take a baking dish and place your parchment paper
3. Cut the goat cheese into round half inch slices
4. Transfer to the baking dish
5. Bake on upper rack until golden
6. Fry the bacon in a pan until they are crispy
7. Cut up the avocados into pieces and place them on top of the arugula
8. Add fried bacon, goat cheese and sprinkle nuts on top
9. Take an immersion blender and make the salad dressing by mixing all the salad ingredients in a bowl and blending them
10. Season with salt and pepper. Dress your salad with the dressing and enjoy!

Nutrition (Per Serving)

- Calories: 592
- Fat: 51g
- Carbohydrates: 12g
- Protein: 22g

Storage Options/Meal Prep Tips: Prepare the ingredients and dressing beforehand. Store them in different zip bags and store in fridge for 2-3

Chapter 13: Breakfast

Amazing Bacon And Cheese Egg Cups

Serving: 6
Prep Time: 10 minutes
Cook Time: 15 minutes
Ingredients

- 6 bacon strips
- 6 large eggs
- Handful of spinach
- ¼ cup cheese
- Salt and pepper to taste

How To

1. Pre-heat your oven to 400 degree F
2. Fry bacon in a skillet over medium heat, drain the oil and keep them on the side
3. Take muffin tin and grease with oil
4. Line with a slice of bacon, press down the bacon well, making sure that the ends are sticking out (to be used as handles)
5. Take a bowl and beat eggs
6. Drain and pat the spinach dry
7. Add the spinach to the eggs
8. Add a quarter of the mixture in each of your muffin tins
9. Sprinkle cheese and season
10. Bake for 15 minutes
11. Enjoy!

Nutrition (Per Serving)

- Calories: 101
- Fat: 7g
- Carbohydrates: 1g
- Protein: 8g

Gently Cinnamon And Coconut Porridge

Serving: 4
Prep Time: 5 minutes
Cook Time: 5 minutes
<u>Ingredients</u>

- 2 cups water
- 1 cup 36% heavy cream
- ½ cup unsweetened dried coconut, shredded
- 2 tablespoons oat bran
- 2 tablespoons flaxseed meal
- 1 tablespoon butter
- 1 and ½ teaspoon stevia
- 1 teaspoon cinnamon
- Salt to taste
- Toppings as blueberries

<u>How To</u>

1. Add the listed ingredients to a small pot, mix well
2. Transfer pot to stove and place it over medium-low heat
3. Bring to mix to a slow boil
4. Stir well and remove the heat
5. Divide the mix into equal servings and let them sit for 10 minutes
6. Top with your desired toppings and enjoy!

<u>Nutrition (Per Serving)</u>

- Calories: 171
- Fat: 16g
- Carbohydrates: 6g
- Protein: 2g

Baked Eggs And Avocado

Serving: 4
Prep Time: 10 minutes
Cook Time: 15 minutes
Ingredients

- 4 whole eggs
- 2 avocados, sliced halved lengthwise and stoned
- Pinch of garlic powder
- Pinch of salt
- Pinch of pepper
- Handful of parmesan cheese, grated

How To

1. Pre-heat your oven to 350 degree F
2. Cut avocado and scoop a quarter of the Avocado flesh
3. Add the flesh to muffin tin
4. Season the avocado halves and crack an egg into each of the halves
5. Sprinkle cheese
6. Place avocado in oven and bake for 15 minutes
7. Take them out and sprinkled scooped avocado flesh on top
8. Serve and enjoy!

Nutrition (Per Serving)

- Calories: 261
- Fat: 20
- Carbohydrates: 3g
- Protein:14g

Smoked Salmon And Cream Cheese Rolls

Serving: 2
Prep Time: 25 minutes
Cook Time: Nil
<u>Ingredients</u>

- 4 ounces cream cheese, at room temperature
- 1 teaspoon grated lemon zest
- 1 teaspoon Dijon mustard
- 2 tablespoons scallions, chopped (white and green parts)
- Pink salt
- Freshly ground black pepper
- 1 pack (4 ounces) cold-smoked salmon (12 slices)

<u>How To</u>

1. Add cream cheese, lemon zest, scallions, mustard in food processor and season with salt and pepper
2. Process until mixed
3. Spread cream –cheese mix on each slice of smoked salmon
4. Roll it up
5. Place rolls on plat (seam side down)
6. Serve and enjoy!

<u>Nutrition (Per Serving)</u>

- Calories: 536
- Fat: 44g
- Carbohydrates: 6g
- Protein: 28g

Satisfying Berry Smoothie

Serving: 1
Prep Time: 4 minutes
Cook Time: Nil
<u>Ingredients</u>

- ¼ cup frozen blueberries
- ¼ cup frozen blackberries
- 1 cup unsweetened almond milk
- 1 teaspoon vanilla bean extract
- 3 teaspoons flaxseed
- 1 scoop chilled Greek yogurt
- Stevia as needed

<u>How To</u>

1. Mix everything in a blender and emulsify them
2. Pulse the mixture four time until you have your desired thickness
3. Pour the mixture into a glass and enjoy!

<u>Nutrition (Per Serving)</u>

- Calories: 221
- Fat: 9g
- Carbohydrates: 8g
- Protein: 21g

Storage Options/Meal Prep Tips: Transfer to mason jars and store in your fridge for 3-4 days.

Hearty Early Morning Cream Cheese Muffins

Serving: 6
Prep Time: 10 minutes
Cook Time: 10 minutes
<u>Ingredients</u>

- 4 tablespoons melted butter, plus more for muffin tin
- 1 cup almond flour
- ¾ tablespoon baking powder
- 2 large eggs, lightly beaten
- 2 ounces cream cheese, mixed with 2 tablespoons heavy cream
- Handful of Mexican blend cheese, shredded

<u>How To</u>

1. Pre-heat your oven to 400 degree F
2. Coat six cups of muffin tin with butter
3. Take a small bowl and add almond flour, baking powder
4. Take a medium bowl and add eggs, cream cheese-heavy cream mix and shredded cheese
5. Add 4 tablespoons of butter
6. Pour flour mix into egg mix and beat using a hand mixer until the mixture is thoroughly mixed
7. Pour batter into muffin cups
8. Bake for 12 minutes until top is golden brown
9. Serve and enjoy!

<u>Nutrition (Per Serving)</u>

- Calories: 247
- Fat: 23g
- Carbohydrates: 4g
- Protein: 8g

Kale And Avocados In A Skillet

Serving: 2
Prep Time: 5 minutes
Cook Time: 10 minutes
<u>Ingredients</u>

- 2 tablespoons olive oil, divided
- 2 cups mushrooms, sliced
- 5 ounces fresh kale, stemmed and sliced into ribbons
- 1 avocado, sliced
- 4 large eggs
- Salt and pepper as needed

<u>How To</u>

1. Take a large skillet and place it over medium heat
2. Add a tablespoon olive oil
3. Add mushrooms to pan and Saute for 3 minutes
4. Take a medium bowl and massage kale with remaining 1 tablespoon olive oil (for about 1-2 minutes)
5. Add kale to skillet and place them on top of mushrooms
6. Place slices of avocado on top of kale
7. Create 4 wells for eggs and crack each egg onto each hold
8. Season eggs with salt and pepper
9. Cover skillet and cook for 5 minutes
10. Serve hot!

<u>Nutrition (Per Serving)</u>

- Calories: 461
- Fat: 34g
- Carbohydrates: 6g
- Protein: 18g

Heart Throb Denver Omelette

Serving: 1
Prep Time: 4 minutes
Cook Time: 1 minute
<u>**Ingredients**</u>

- 2 tablespoons butter
- ¼ cup onion, chopped
- ¼ cup green bell pepper, diced
- ¼ cup grape tomatoes, halved
- 2 whole eggs
- ¼ cup ham, chopped

<u>**How To**</u>

1. Take a skillet and place it over medium heat
2. Add butter and wait until the butter melts
3. Add onion and bell pepper and Saute for a few minutes
4. Take a bowl and whip eggs
5. Add the remaining ingredients and stir
6. Add Sautéed onion and pepper, stir
7. Microwave the egg mix for 1 minute
8. Serve hot!

<u>**Nutrition (Per Serving)**</u>

- Calories: 605
- Fat: 946g
- Carbohydrates: 6g
- Protein: 39g

Fascinating Pork Frittata

Serving: 4
Prep Time: 5 minutes
Cook Time: 25 minutes
<u>Ingredients</u>

- 1 tablespoons butter
- 8 large eggs
- 1 cup heavy cream
- Pink salt
- Freshly ground black pepper
- 4 ounces pancetta, chopped
- 2 ounces prosciutto, thinly sliced
- 1 tablespoon fresh dill, chopped

<u>How To</u>

1. Pre-heat your oven to 375 degree F
2. Coat a 9 by 13 inch baking pan and grease with butter
3. Take a large bowl and whisk in eggs, cream and season with salt and pepper
4. Whisk well
5. Pour egg mix into prepped pans and sprinkle pancetta
6. Distribute evenly
7. Tear off pieces of prosciutto and place on top
8. Sprinkle dill
9. Bake for 25 minutes until edges are golden
10. Transfer to cooling rack and let it sit for 5 minutes
11. Cut into 4 portions, serve and enjoy!

<u>Nutrition (Per Serving)</u>

- Calories: 437
- Fat: 39g
- Carbohydrates: 3g
- Protein: 21g

Early Morning Green Smoothie

Serving: 3
Prep Time: 10 minutes
Cook Time: Nil
<u>Ingredients</u>

- ½ a avocado, pitted and peeled
- 7 ounces full fat unsweetened coconut milk
- 1 cup baby kale, chopped
- ½ cup cucumber, diced
- 2 tablespoons freshly squeezed lemon juice
- 2 tablespoons fresh squeezed orange juice
- Water as needed

<u>How To</u>

1. Add the listed ingredients to your blender
2. Blend on low until mixed
3. Increase the mixer power to high and blend until you have a smooth texture
4. Add a few drops of stevia for extra taste
5. Divide the mix into 3 servings and enjoy!

<u>Nutrition (Per Serving)</u>

- Calories: 218
- Fat: 21g
- Carbohydrates: 9g
- Protein: 3g

Chapter 14: Lunch and Dinner

Generous Tomato And Basil Soup

Serving: 6
Prep Time: 10 minutes
Cook Time: 25 minutes
<u>Ingredients</u>

- 2 tablespoons olive oil
- 1 yellow onion, diced
- 2 garlic cloves, minced
- 2 cans (28 ounces) whole peeled tomatoes, with juice
- 2 cups vegetable broth
- ½ cup salted butter
- ½ cup basil leaves, chopped
- 1 cup heavy whipping cream
- Salt and pepper as needed

<u>How To</u>

1. Take a large stock pot and place it over medium heat
2. Add olive oil and heat up
3. Add onion, garlic and cook for 5 minutes until browned
4. Add tomatoes with juice, broth and butter, bring the mix to a boil
5. Lower down heat to low, simmer uncovered for 20 minutes
6. Add basil and puree the soup using immersion blender
7. Stir in cream
8. Season with salt and pepper and serve. Enjoy!

<u>Nutrition (Per Serving)</u>

- Calories: 371
- Fat: 36g
- Carbohydrates: 9g
- Protein: 4g

Storage Options/Meal Prep Tips: Transfer to air tight containers and seal tightly. Store in fridge for 2-3 days and in freezer for 2-3 months.

Fantastic Garlic And Butter Cod

Serving: 3
Prep Time: 5 minutes
Cook Time: 20 minutes
<u>**Ingredients**</u>

- 3 cod fillets, 8 ounces each
- ¾ pound baby bok choy, halved
- 1/3 cup butter, thinly sliced
- 1 and ½ tablespoons garlic, minced
- Salt and pepper to taste

<u>**How To**</u>

1. Pre-heat your oven to 400 degree F
2. Cut 3 sheets of aluminum foil (large enough to fit fillet)
3. Place cod fillet on each sheet and add butter and garlic on top
4. Add bok choy, season with pepper and salt
5. Fold packet and enclose them in pouches
6. Arrange on baking sheet
7. Bake for 20 minutes
8. Transfer to cooling rack and let them cool
9. Enjoy!

<u>**Nutrition (Per Serving)**</u>

- Calories: 355
- Fat: 21g
- Carbohydrates: 3g
- Protein: 37g

Storage Options/Meal Prep Tips: Store in airtight containers and refrigerate for up to 3 days. Make sure to re-heat in oven before serving.   Freezer time 4-6 months.

Garlic And Parsley Chicken Feast

Serving: 4
Prep Time: 10 minutes
Cook Time: 40 minutes
<u>Ingredients</u>

- 1 tablespoon dry parsley
- 1 tablespoon dry basil
- 4 chicken breast halves, boneless and skinless
- ½ teaspoon salt
- ½ teaspoon red pepper flakes, crushed
- 2 tomatoes, sliced

<u>How To</u>

1. Pre-heat your oven to 350 degree F
2. Take a 9x13 inch baking dish and grease it up with cooking spray
3. Sprinkle 1 tablespoon of parsley, 1 teaspoon of basil and spread the mixture over your baking dish
4. Arrange the chicken breast halves over the dish and sprinkle garlic slices on top
5. Take a small bowl and add 1 teaspoon parsley, 1 teaspoon of basil, salt, basil, red pepper and mix well. Pour the mixture over the chicken breast
6. Top with tomato slices and cover, bake for 25 minutes
7. Remove the cover and bake for 15 minutes more
8. Serve and enjoy!

<u>Nutrition (Per Serving)</u>

- Calories: 150
- Fat: 4g
- Carbohydrates: 4g
- Protein: 25g

Storage Options/Meal Prep Tips: Transfer to air tight containers and seal tightly. Store in fridge for 2-3 days and in freezer for 2-3 months.

Delicious Broccoli Tilapia

Serving: 2
Prep Time: 4 minutes
Cook Time: 14 minutes
Ingredients

- 6 ounce of tilapia, frozen
- 1 tablespoon of butter
- 1 tablespoon of garlic, minced
- 1 teaspoon of lemon pepper seasoning
- 1 cup of broccoli florets, fresh

How To

1. Pre-heat your oven to 350 degree F
2. Add fish in aluminum foil packets
3. Arrange broccoli around fish
4. Sprinkle lemon pepper on top
5. Close the packets and seal
6. Bake for 14 minutes
7. Take a bowl and add garlic and butter, mix well and keep the mixture on the side
8. Remove the packet from oven and transfer to platter
9. Place butter on top of the fish and broccoli, serve and enjoy!

Nutrition (Per Serving)

- Calories: 362
- Fat: 25g
- Carbohydrates: 2g
- Protein: 29g

Storage Options/Meal Prep Tips: You may prep the ingredients beforehand by add butter and garlic into a small zip bags and the cut broccoli in another zip bag. As for the lemon pepper, simply keep them in a small container. Freezer time 4-6 months.

Cool Balsamic Chicken And Veggies

Serving: 4
Prep Time: 15 minutes
Cook Time: 25 minutes
<u>**Ingredients**</u>

- 8 chickne thigh, boneless and skinless
- 10 stalks asparagus, halved
- 2 peppers, cut in chunks
- 1 red onion, diced
- ½ cup carrots, sliced
- 2 garlic cloves, minced
- 5 ounces mushrooms, diced
- ¼ cup baslamic vinegar
- 2 tablespoons olive oil
- ½ teaspoon stevia
- ½ tablespoon oregano
- Salt and pepper to taste

How To

1. Pre-heat your oven to 425 degree F
2. Take a bowl and add all of the vegetables and mix
3. Add spices and oil and mix
4. Dip the chicken pieces into spice mix and coat them well
5. Place the veggies and chicken onto a pan in a single layer
6. Cook for 25 minutes
7. Serve and enjoy!

Nutrition (Per Serving)

- Calories: 362
- Fat: 25g
- Carbohydrates: 2g
- Protein: 29g

Storage Options/Meal Prep Tips: You may prep the ingredients beforehand by add butter and garlic into a small zip bags and the cut broccoli in another zip bag. As for the lemon pepper, simply keep them in a small container. Freezer time 4-6 months

Fine Rotisserie Chicken With Shredded Cabbage

Serving: 2
Prep Time: 5 minutes
Cook Time: Nil
<u>Ingredients</u>

- 1 pound rotisserie chicken, cooked
- 7 ounces frsh green cabbage
- ½ a red onion
- 1 tablespoon olive oil
- ½ cup Keto-Friendly mayonnaise
- Salt and pepper to taste

<u>How To</u>

1. Shred cabbage using a sharp knife and place them on a plate
2. Slice onion thinly and add them to the plate
3. Add rotisserie chicken to the plate and add mayonnaise
4. Drizzle olive oil
5. Season with salt and pepper
6. Mix well and enjoy!

<u>Nutrition (Per Serving)</u>

- Calories: 423
- Fat: 35g
- Carbohydrates: 6g
- Protein: 17g

Storage Options/Meal Prep Tips: Transfer to air tight containers and seal tightly. Store in fridge for 2-3 days and in freezer for 2-3 months.

Fantastic Asian Beef Steak

Serving: 2
Prep Time: 4 minutes
Cook Time: 4 minutes
<u>Ingredients</u>

- 2 tablespoon of sriracha sauce
- 1 tablespoon of garlic, minced
- 1 tablespoon of ginger, freshly grated
- 1 yellow bell pepper, cut in strips
- 1 red bell pepper cut in thin strips
- 1 tablespoon of sesame oil, garlic flavored
- 1 tablespoon of stevia
- ½ a teaspoon of curry powder
- ½ a teaspoon of rice wine vinegar
- 8 ounce of beef sirloin cut into strips
- 2 cups of baby spinach, stemmed
- ½ head of butter of lettuce, torn

<u>How To</u>

1. Add garlic, sriracha sauce, 1 teaspoon of sesame oil, rice wine vinegar and stevia bowl
2. Mix well
3. Pour half of the mix into zip bag and add steak, allow it to marinade
4. Assemble the brightly colored salad by layer the vegetables in two bowls in the following order: baby spinach, butter lettuce, two peppers on top
5. Remove the steak from marinade and discard the liquid
6. Heat up sesame oil in skillet over medium heat and add steak, stir fry for 3 minutes Transfer your cooker steak on top of the salad
7. Drizzle the other half of your marinade mix
8. Sprinkle sriracha sauce on top and serve!

<u>Nutrition (Per Serving)</u>

- Calories: 350
- Fat: 23g
- Carbohydrates: 4g
- Protein: 28g

Storage Options/Meal Prep Tips: It is possible to store the salad and steak individual in zip bags in your refrigerator and serve by assembling them. Make sure to not exceed 2-3 days of refrigeration time. Freezer time 3-4 months.

Juicy Steak And Broccoli Delight

Serving: 4
Prep Time: 5 minutes
Cook Time: 15 minutes
Ingredients

- 4 ounces butter
- ¾ pound Ribeye steak, sliced
- 9 ounces broccoli, chopped
- 1 yellow onion, sliced
- 1 tablespoon coconut aminos
- 1 tablespoon pumpkin seeds
- Salt and pepper to taste

How To

1. Slice steak and onions
2. Chop broccoli (including the stems)
3. Take a frying pan and heat it over medium-heat
4. Add butter and let it melt
5. Add meat and season with salt and pepper
6. Cook until both sides are browned (or cooked to your desired doneness)
7. Transfer the meat to a platter
8. Add broccoli and onion, add more butter
9. Brown them
10. Add coconut aminos and return the meat
11. Stir and season
12. Serve with a dollop of butter and pumpkin seeds Enjoy!

Nutrition (Per Serving)

- Calories: 875
- Fat: 75g
- Carbohydrates: 10g
- Protein: 40g

Storage Options/Meal Prep Tips: Transfer to airtight container and refrigerate for 2-3 days at max. Serve by re-heating and adding a dollop of butter. Freezer time 3-4 months.

Magical Cucumber Soup

Serving: 4
Prep Time: 14 minutes
Cook Time: Nil
<u>**Ingredients**</u>

- 2 tablespoons garlic, minced
- 4 cups english cucumbers, peeled and diced
- ½ cup onions, diced
- 1 tablespoon lemon juice
- 1 and ½ cups vegetable broth
- ½ teaspoon salt
- ¼ teaspoon red pepper flakes
- ¼ cup parsley, diced
- ½ cup Greek yogurt, plain

<u>**How To**</u>

6. Add the listed ingredients to blender and emulsify by blend them (except ½ cup of chopped cucumbers)
7. Blend until smooth
8. Divide the soup amongst 4 servings and top with extra cucumbers
9. Enjoy chilled!

<u>**Nutrition (Per Serving)**</u>

- Calories: 169
- Fat: 12g
- Carbohydrates: 6g
- Protein: 4g

Storage Options/Meal Prep Tips: Freeze the servings in individual containers with lids. Microwave before serving. Freezer time 2-3 months.

Simple Parmesan Baked Chicken

Serving: 2
Prep Time: 5 minutes
Cook Time: 20 minutes
Ingredients

- 2 tablespoons ghee
- 2 boneless chicken breasts, skinless
- Pink salt
- Freshly ground black pepper
- ½ cup mayonnaise
- ¼ cup parmesan cheese, grated
- 1 tablespoon dried Italian seasoning
- ¼ cup crushed pork rinds

How To

1. Pre-heat your oven to 425 degree F
2. Take a large baking dish and coat with ghee
3. Pat chicken breasts dry and wrap with towel
4. Season with salt and pepper
5. Place in baking dish
6. Take a small bowl and add mayonnaise, parmesan cheese, Italian seasoning
7. Slather mayo mix evenly over chicken breast
8. Sprinkle crushed pork rinds on top
9. Bake for 20 minutes until topping is browned
10. Serve and enjoy!

Nutrition (Per Serving)

- Calories: 850
- Fat: 67g
- Carbohydrates: 2g
- Protein: 60g

Storage Options/Meal Prep Tips: Transfer to air tight containers and seal tightly. Store in fridge for 2-3 days and in freezer for 2-3 months.

Chapter 15: Sides

Crispy Walnut Bites

Serving: 10
Prep Time: 10 minutes
Cook Time: 8 minutes
<u>Ingredients</u>

- 6 ounces parmesan cheese, grated
- 2 tablespoons walnuts, chopped
- 1 tablespoons unsalted butter
- ½ tablespoon fresh thyme chopped

<u>How To</u>

1. Pre-heat your oven to 350 degree F
2. Take two large rimmed baking sheets and line with parchment
3. Add cheese, butter to food processor and blend
4. Add walnuts to the mix and pulse
5. Take a tablespoon and scoop mix onto baking sheet
6. Top with chopped thymes
7. Bake for 8 minutes, transfer to cooling rack
8. Let it cool for 30 minutes
9. Serve and enjoy!

<u>Nutrition (Per Serving)</u>

- Calories: 80
- Fat: 3g
- Carbohydrates: 7g
- Protein: 7g

Storage Options/Meal Prep Tips: Store in airtight container and serve when needed, refrigerate for up to 5 days. Freezer time 2-3 months.

The Very Low-Carb Cheese Omelette

Serving: 5
Prep Time: 5 minutes
Cook Time: 5 minutes
<u>Ingredients</u>

- 2 whole eggs
- 1 tablespoon water
- 1 tablespoon butter
- 3 thin slices salami
- 5 fresh basil leaves
- 5 thin slices, fresh ripe tomatoes
- 2 ounces fresh mozarella cheese
- Salt and pepper as needed

<u>How To</u>

1. Whisk eggs and water in a small bowl and mix well
2. Place a non-stick Saute pan over medium-low heat and melt butter
3. Pour the egg mix and cook for 30 seconds
4. Spread the Salami slices on one half of the egg mix
5. Top with cheese, tomatoes, basil slices and season with pepper and salt
6. Cook for 2 minutes and the empty half of the egg is firm to be folded, use a spatula to fold the Omelette in half
7. Cover and cook on LOW heat for 1 minute
8. Remove and enjoy!

<u>Nutrition (Per Serving)</u>

- Calories: 451
- Fat: 36g
- Carbohydrates: 3g
- Protein: 33g

Supreme Chocolate-Avocado Pudding

Serving: 2
Prep Time: 5 minutes + 30 chill time
Cook Time: Nil
<u>Ingredients</u>

- 1 ripe medium avocado, cut into chunks
- 2 ounces cream cheese, at room temperature
- 1 tablespoon Swerve natural sweetener
- 4 tablespoons Unsweetened cocoa powder
- ¼ teaspoon vanilla extract
- Pink salt as needed

<u>How To</u>

1. Take a food processor and add avocado, cream cheese, sweetener, cocoa powder, salt and vanilla
2. Blend until smooth
3. Pour into dessert bowls
4. Chill for 30 minutes and serve
5. Enjoy!

<u>Nutrition (Per Serving)</u>

- Calories: 80
- Fat: 3g
- Carbohydrates: 7g
- Protein: 7g

Cool Mascarpone And Pecan Bowl

Serving: 2
Prep Time: 5 minutes
Cook Time: Nil
<u>Ingredients</u>

- 1 cup chopped pecans
- 1 drop liquid stevia
- ¼ cup mascarpone
- 30 Lily's dark chocolate chips
- 6 strawberries, sliced

<u>How To</u>

1. Divide the pecans between dessert bowls
2. Take a small bowl and add sweetener and mascarpone cheese
3. Take serving bowl and add nuts
4. Top with a dollop of sweetened mascarpone
5. Sprinkle chocolate chips and top with strawberries
6. Enjoy!

<u>Nutrition (Per Serving)</u>

- Calories: 462
- Fat: 47g
- Carbohydrates: 6g
- Protein: 6g

Storage Options/Meal Prep Tips: Transfer to air tight containers and seal tightly. Store in fridge for 7 days.

Grilled Artichoke Bites

Serving: 6
Prep Time: 5 minutes
Cook Time: 30 minutes
Ingredients

- 2 large artichokes
- 1 lemon, quartered
- ¾ cup olive oil
- 4 garlic cloves, chopped
- 1 teaspoon salt
- ½ teaspoon black pepper

How To

1. Take a large sized bowl and add water
2. Squeeze lemon juice in the water
3. Trim the top of the artichokes and cut them half-lengthwise
4. Bring the water to a boil and add the artichokes, allow them to cook for 15 minutes
5. While they are being cooked, pre-heat your grill to medium-high
6. Once the chokes are cooked, drain them and squeeze the rest of the lemon wedges into a medium sized bowl
7. Stir in garlic and olive oil
8. Season with pepper and salt
9. Brush the chokes with the coating of garlic dip and place them on the pre-heated grill
10. Grill for 10 minutes, makings sure to keep basting it from time to time
11. Serve the grilled artichokes with the rest of the dips

Nutrition (Per Serving)

- Calories: 237
- Fat: 19g
- Carbohydrates: 12g
- Protein: 5g

Storage Options/Meal Prep Tips: Store the servings in airtight containers for about 2-3 days.

Subtle Salmon Stuffed Avocado

Serving: 2
Prep Time: 10 minutes
Cook Time: 30 minutes
<u>Ingredients</u>

- 1 ripe oragnic avocado
- 2 ounces wild caught smoked salmon
- 1 ounce fresh goat cheese
- 2 tablespoons extra virgin olive oil
- Salt as needed

<u>How To</u>

1. Cut up the avocado in two and deseed
2. Take a small food processor and add remaining ingredients and mix well until coarsely chopped up
3. Place the mixture into the avocado
4. Serve immediately and enjoy!

<u>Nutrition (Per Serving)</u>

- Calories: 525
- Fat: 48g
- Carbohydrates: 4g
- Protein: 19g

Storage Options/Meal Prep Tips: Transfer to air tight containers and seal tightly. Store in fridge for 2-3 days and in freezer for 2-3 months.

Lemon And Broccoli Awesome Platter

Serving: 6
Prep Time: 10 minutes
Cook Time: 15 minutes

Ingredients

- 2 heads brococli, separated into florets
- 2 teaspoons extra virgin olive oil
- 1 teaspoon salt
- ½ teaspoon black pepper
- 1 garlic clove, minced
- ½ teaspoon lemon juice

How To

1. Pre-heat your oven to a temperature of 400 degree F
2. Take a large sized bowl and add broccoli florets with some extra virgin olive oil, pepper, sea salt and garlic
3. Spread the broccoli out in a single even layer on a fine baking sheet
4. Bake in your pre-heated oven for about 15-20 minutes until the florets are soft enough so that they can be pierced with a fork
5. Squeeze lemon juice over them generously before serving
6. Enjoy!

Nutrition (Per Serving)

- Calories: 49
- Fat: 1.9g
- Carbohydrates: 7g
- Protein: 3g

Storage Options/Meal Prep Tips: Transfer to air tight containers and seal tightly. Store in fridge for 2-3 days and in freezer for 2-3 months.

Sautéed Zucchini Bites

Serving: 6
Prep Time: 5 minutes
Cook Time: 30 minutes
<u>Ingredients</u>

- 1 tablespoon olive oil
- ½ red onion, diced
- Salt and pepper to taste
- 4 zucchini, halved and sliced
- ½ pound fresh mushroom, sliced
- 1 tomato, diced
- 1 garlic clove, minced
- 1 teapsoon Italian seasoning

<u>How To</u>

1. Take a large skillet and place it over medium heat
2. Add onion and Saute for 2 minutes
3. Season with salt and pepper
4. Add zucchini to skillet, cook until tender
5. Add garlic, Italian seasoning and tomatoes
6. Cook and enjoy!

<u>Nutrition (Per Serving)</u>

- Calories: 230
- Fat: 22g
- Carbohydrates: 4g
- Protein: 5g

Storage Options/Meal Prep Tips: Store the servings in airtight containers for about 2-3 days.

Cool Pesto Scrambled Eggs

Serving: 5
Prep Time: 5 minutes
Cook Time: 5 minutes
<u>Ingredients</u>

- 3 large whole eggs
- 1 tablespoon butter
- 1 tablespoon pesto
- 2 tablespoons creamed coconut milk
- Salt and pepper as needed

<u>How To</u>

1. Crack eggs into a bowl and add a pinch of salt and pepper
2. Beat well
3. Pour the eggs into a pan and add butter
4. Turn the heat on
5. Keep cooking on low and gently add the pesto
6. Remove the heat and spoon in coconut cream and mix well
7. Cook for a while and remove the heat once you have a creamy texture
8. Serve and enjoy with Keto buns!

<u>Nutrition (Per Serving)</u>

- Calories: 467
- Fat: 41g
- Carbohydrates: 3g
- Protein: 20g

Crustless Cheesecake Bites

Serving: 4
Prep Time: 10 minutes + 3 hours chill time
Cook Time: 30 minutes
<u>Ingredients</u>

- 4 ounces cream cheese, at room temperature
- ¼ cup sour cream
- 2 whole large eggs
- ¼ cup Swerve
- ¼ teaspoon vanilla extract

<u>How To</u>

1. Pre-heat your oven to 350 degree F
2. Take a medium mixing bowl and add cream cheese, eggs, sour cream, sweetener, vanilla and beat using hand mixer
3. Place cupcake liner in muffin tins
4. Pour cheesecake batters into liners and bake for 30 minutes
5. Let them chill for 3 hours
6. Serve and enjoy!

<u>Nutrition (Per Serving)</u>

- Calories: 677
- Fat: 60g
- Carbohydrates: 7g
- Protein: 20g

Chapter 16: Sweet Treats

Subtle Keto Hot Fudge

Serving: 10
Prep Time: 5 minutes
Cook Time: 10 minutes
<u>Ingredients</u>

- ½ cup salted butter
- 4 ounces dark chocolate
- 2 tablespoons unsweetened cocoa powder
- 1 cup swerve
- 1 cup heavy whipping cream
- 2 teaspoons vanilla extract
- Pinch of salt

<u>How To</u>

1. Take a medium saucepan and place it over medium heat
2. Add butter and chocolate and melt
3. Add cocoa powder and sweetener
4. Whisk for 3-5 minutes until everything dissolves
5. Add cream and bring to a boil
6. Stir
7. Lower down heat to low and add vanilla and salt
8. Remove heat
9. Let it sit for 5 minutes
10. Serve hot and enjoy!

<u>Nutrition (Per Serving)</u>

- Calories: 237
- Fat: 24g
- Carbohydrates: 3g
- Protein: 2g

Simple 5 Minute Chocolate Mousse

Serving: 4
Prep Time: 5 minutes
Cook Time: Nil
<u>Ingredients</u>

- 1 can (14.5 ounces) coconut cream, chilled
- 3 tablespoons unsweetened cocoa powder
- ¼ cup Swerve
- 1 teaspoon vanilla extract

<u>How To</u>

1. Take a large mixing bowl whip in coconut cream with hand mixer, keep whipping for 3 minutes until fluffy
2. Fold in cocoa powder, swerve, vanilla and serve immediately
3. Enjoy!

<u>Nutrition (Per Serving)</u>

- Calories: 222
- Fat: 22g
- Carbohydrates: 4g
- Protein: 1g

Chocolate Chip Cookie In A Skillet

Serving: 8
Prep Time: 10 minutes + 10 minutes resting time
Cook Time: 25 minutes
Ingredients

- Olive oil for coking
- 1 cup almond flour
- ½ cup coconut flour
- ½ teaspoon baking soda
- 1 teaspoon salt
- ½ cup coconut oil
- ¼ cup Swerve
- 1 large egg
- 1 teaspoon vanilla extract
- 1 cup sugar-free chocolate chips

How To

1. Pre-heat your oven to 350 degree F
2. Spray a 9-inch cast iron skillet with cooking spray/ grease with coconut oil
3. Take a large bowl and whisk in almond flour, coconut flour, baking soda, salt
4. Add coconut, oil, swerve, egg, vanilla and whisk until combined
5. Fold in chocolate chips
6. Pour batter into prepped skillet and bake for 20-25 minutes, until edges are browned
7. Let them rest for 10 minutes and serve warm
8. Enjoy!

Nutrition (Per Serving)

- Calories: 390
- Fat: 30g
- Carbohydrates: 20g
- Protein: 7g

Storage Options/Meal Prep Tips: Transfer to air tight containers and seal tightly. Store in fridge for 7 days.

Hearty Peanut Butter Fat Bombs

Serving: 10
Prep Time: 15 minutes + 4 hours freeze time
Cook Time: 1 minute
Ingredients

- 2 tablespoons coconut oil
- 2 tablespoons salted butter
- ¼ cup peanut butter
- ¼ cup swerve
- 2 teaspoons vanilla extract
- 2 tablespoons cream cheese

How To

1. Take a medium sized microwave-safe bowl and add coconut oil, peanut butter, butter, swerve, vanilla, cream cheese and Microwave in increments of 15 seconds, making sure to stir after every 15 seconds session
2. Pour the mixture into ice cube tray and freeze for at least 4 hours
3. Remove from molds and store in air tight containers
4. Serve and enjoy!

Nutrition (Per Serving)

- Calories: 94
- Fat: 9g
- Carbohydrates: 0g
- Protein: 2g

Storage Options/Meal Prep Tips: Transfer to air tight containers and seal tightly. Store in fridge for 7 days.

Awesome Orange Cream Float

Serving: 2
Prep Time: 5 minutes
Cook Time: Nil
<u>Ingredients</u>

- 1 can diet orange soda, such as Zevia's
- 4 tablespoons heavy cream
- 1 teaspoon vanilla extract
- 6 ice cubes

<u>How To</u>

1. Add orange soda, vanilla, ice and cream to your food processor
2. Blend well and pour into tall glasses
3. Serve chilled and enjoy!

<u>Nutrition (Per Serving)</u>

- Calories: 56
- Fat: 6g
- Carbohydrates: 1g
- Protein: 1g

Choco Coated Bacons

Serving: 6
Prep Time: 15 minutes
Cook Time: 20 minutes
<u>Ingredients</u>

- 12 bacon slices
- 4 and ½ tablespoons unsweetened dark chocolate
- 2 and ¼ tablespoons coconut oil
- 1 and ½ teaspoons liquid stevia

<u>How To</u>

1. Pre-heat your oven to 425 degree F
2. Skewer bacon into iron skewers
3. Arrange skewers on a baking sheet and bake for 15 minutes until crispy
4. Transfer to cooling rack
5. Take a saucepan and place it over low heat, add coconut oil and let it melt
6. Stir in chocolate until it melts
7. Add stevia and stir
8. Place crispy bacon on a sheet of parchment paper and drizzle the chocolate mix over
9. Let the chocolate dry
10. Serve an enjoy!

<u>Nutrition (Per Serving)</u>

- Calories:258
- Fat: 26g
- Carbohydrates: 0.5g
- Protein: 7g

Storage Options/Meal Prep Tips: Transfer to airtight containers and serve when needed, possible to refrigerate for 5 days.

The Best Caramel Almond Bars

Serving: 12
Prep Time: 10 minutes + 10 minutes rest time
Cook Time: 20 minute
<u>**Ingredients**</u>

- 2 tablespoons coconut oil
- 6 tablespoons salted butter, melted
- 1 cup unsweetened flaked coconut
- 1 cup almonds, sliced
- ¾ cup almond flour
- ½ cup swerve
- 1 teaspoon salt
- ½ teaspoon baking soda
- 1 cup sugar-free chocolate chips
- 1 cup hot caramel sauce

<u>**How To**</u>

1. Pre-heat your oven to 350 degree F
2. Grease a square baking dish with butter
3. Take a food processor and add coconut, almonds, almond flour, swerve, salt, baking soda and 6 tablespoons of melted butter
4. Pulse until crumbly
5. Fold in chocolate chips and press batter into prepped baking dish
6. Bake for 15-20 minutes until golden brown
7. Pour caramel sauce over bars
8. Let them rest for 10 minutes
9. Serve warm and enjoy!

<u>**Nutrition (Per Serving)**</u>

- Calories: 229
- Fat: 21g
- Carbohydrates: 4g
- Protein: 3g

Storage Options/Meal Prep Tips: Transfer to air tight containers and seal tightly. Store in fridge for 7 days.

Raspberry And Cheese Pops

Serving: 8
Prep Time: 20 minutes
Cook Time: Nil
<u>Ingredients</u>

- ¼ cup cream cheese
- ¼ cup fresh raspberries, chopped
- 4 tablespoons coconut oil
- 4 tablespoons heavy cream
- 4 tablespoons butter
- 1 teaspoon pura vanilla bean extract

<u>How To</u>

1. Add cream cheese, coconut oil, butter in a bowl
2. Mix well and microwave in 10 seconds interval until the cheese has melted
3. Remove the bowl and stir
4. Stir in heavy cream and fold in chopped raspberries
5. Stir in vanilla extra into the mix and stir
6. Pour the mix into ice cube tray for 16 sections Chill for 2 hours and serve!

<u>Nutrition (Per Serving)</u>

- Calories: 166
- Fat: 17g
- Carbohydrates: 2g
- Protein: 0.8g

Storage Options/Meal Prep Tips: Can be stored in refrigerator for at best 2 weeks!

Fancy Blackberry Chia Pudding

Serving: 2
Prep Time: 10 minutes + overnight setting time
Cook Time: Nil
<u>Ingredients</u>

- 1 cup unsweetened full-fat coconut milk
- 1 teaspoon liquid stevia
- 1 teaspoon vanilla extract
- ½ cup blackberries, fresh or frozen
- ¼ cup chia seeds

<u>How To</u>

1. Take a food processor and add coconut milk, vanilla, stevia and mix until thick
2. Add blackberries and process and mixed
3. Fold in chia seeds
4. Divide the mix between small cups and let it sit in your fridge overnight
5. Serve and enjoy!

<u>Nutrition (Per Serving)</u>

- Calories: 873
- Fat: 75g
- Carbohydrates: 15g
- Protein: 15g

Strawberry And Lime Pops

Serving: 4
Prep Time: 5 minutes + 2 hours freezing
Cook Time: Nil
<u>Ingredients</u>

- ½ can (13.5 ounces) coconut cream
- 2 teaspoons Swerve
- 1 tablespoon freshly squeezed lime juice
- ¼ cup hulled and sliced strwaberries

<u>How To</u>

1. Take a food processor and add coconut cream, lime juice and sweetener
2. Add strawberries, pulse for a few times (the strawberries should maintain their texture)
3. Pour into ice pop molds
4. Freeze for 2 hours
5. Serve!

<u>Nutrition (Per Serving)</u>

- Calories: 166
- Fat: 17g
- Carbohydrates: 3g
- Protein: 1g

Conclusion

I would like to thank you for purchasing the book and taking the time for going through the book as well.

I do hope that this book has been helpful and you found the information contained within the scriptures useful!

Keep in mind that you are not only limited to the recipes provided in this book! Just go ahead and keep on exploring until find the perfect recipes for your Ketogenic journey!

Stay healthy and stay safe!

Appendix

Volume Equivalents (Liquid)

US STANDARD	US STANDARD (OUNCES)	METRIC (APPROXIMATE)
2 tablespoons	1 fl. oz.	30 mL
¼ cup	2 fl. oz.	60 mL
½ cup	4 fl. oz.	120 mL
1 cup	8 fl. oz.	240 mL
1 and ½ cups	12 fl. oz.	355 mL
2 cups/ 1 pint	16 fl. oz.	475 mL
4 cups/ 1 quart	32 fl. oz.	1 L
1 gallon	128 fl. oz.	4 L

Volume Equivalents (Dry)

US STANDARD	METRIC (APPROXIMATE)
¼ teaspoon	1 mL
½ teaspoon	2 mL
1 teaspoon	5 mL
1 tablespoon	15 mL
¼ cup	59 mL
½ cup	118 mL
1 cup	177 L

Oven Temperatures

FAHRENHEIT (°F)	CELSIUS (°C) (APPROXIMATE)
250 °F	120 °C
300 °F	150 °C
325 °F	165 °C
350 °F	180 °C
375 °F	190 °C
400 °F	200 °C
425 °F	220 °C
450 °F	230 °F

Weight Equivalents

US STANDARD	METRIC (APPROXIMATE)
½ ounce	15 g
1 ounce	30 g
2 ounces	60 g
4 ounces	115 g
8 ounces	225 g
12 ounces	340 g
16 ounces/1 pound	455 g